Trauma and Pain in Wound Care

edited by
Richard White and Keith Harding

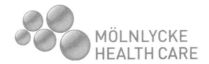

MÖLNLYCKE
HEALTH CARE

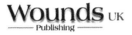

Wounds UK
Publishing

Wounds UK Publishing, Wounds UK Limited, Suite 3.1, 36 Upperkirkgate,
Aberdeen AB10 1BA

British Library Cataloguing-in-Publication Data
A catalogue record is available for this book

ISBN 0-9549193-7-8

Printed in the UK by Cromwell Press, Trowbridge, Wiltshire

CONTENTS

Section III: Aspects of wound trauma and pain

LIST OF CONTRIBUTORS

Pauline Beldon is Tissue Viability Nurse Consultant, Epsom and St Helier University Hospitals NHS Trust, Carshalton.

Janice Cameron is an Independent Nurse Advisor in Wound Care, Witney, Oxfordshire.

Pam Cooper is Clinical Nurse Specialist in Tissue Viability, Department of Tissue Viability, Grampian NHS Acute Trust, Aberdeen.

Dr Valentina Dini is Consultant Dermatologist, Department of Dermatology, University of Pisa.

Valerie Douglas is Lecturer Practitioner in Tissue Viability for Bournemouth Teaching PCT and Bournemouth University.

David Gray is Clinical Director of Wounds UK and a Clinical Nurse Specialist in the Elderly Medicine and Continuing Care Psychiatric Units, Department of Tissue Viability, Grampian NHS Acute Trust, Aberdeen.

Keith Harding is Departmental Head of the Wound Healing Research Unit, School of Medicine, Cardiff University and Clinical Director of Wound Healing in the Cardiff and Vale NHS Trust.

Deborah Hofman is Clinical Nurse Specialist, Wound Healing, and Lead Nurse, Leg Ulcer Clinic, Department of Dermatology, Churchill Hospital, Oxford.

Helen Hollinworth is Senior Teaching Practitioner, Faculty of Health, Suffolk College, Ipswich.

Mark Johnson is Professor of Pain and Analgesia, Leeds Metropolitan University.

Adam Katchky is a Medical Student at Dermatology Daycare and Wound Healing Clinic, Sunnybrook, Ontario, Canada.

Patricia Price is Professor of Health Sciences, Wound Healing Research Unit, Cardiff University.

Douglas Queen is Business Consultant at Toronto Wound Healing Centres, Toronto, Canada and Editor of the *International Wound Journal*.

Professor Marco Romanelli is Director, Wound Healing Research Unit, University of Pisa.

R Gary Sibbald is Professor, Medicine and Public Health Science; Director of Continuing Education, Department of Medicine, University of Toronto; Director of Dermatology, Daycare and Wound Healing Clinic, Sunnybrook and Women's Health Sciences Centre; Toronto Wound Healing Centres, Toronto, Ontario; and Chairman (Toronto Meeting 2008) of the World Union of Wound Healing Societies.

Richard White is a Clinical Research Consultant and Senior Research Fellow, Department of Tissue Viability, Aberdeen Royal Infirmary.

FOREWORD

Wound healing as a specialty is still in its infancy. Since the advent of moist wound healing the goal of treatment has almost exclusively been focused on complete healing. In recent years, as a reflection of increasing maturity, it has been recognised that alternative treatment goals are not only desirable, but also essential. Of the many advances made in wound management in recent years, few will have as much impact as the trend towards 'patient-centred care' as recognising the importance of pain. This is based upon quality of life aspects relevant to the individual with a wound. A key component of this trend is the recognition of wound-related pain, its assessment, and strategies to avoid or manage. The focus on pain has resulted in seminal guidelines and best practice statements from the World Union of Wound Healing Societies (WUWHS), the European Wound Management Association (EWMA), and the Independent Advisory Group. Each of these is referenced throughout this book, and, attention is given to each in a review chapter at the end of this book.

The theme of this book is wound trauma and pain. It is intended to develop and increase awareness of wound pain, trauma in wound management-related procedures, and the patient-centred approaches that these measures demand.

Each chapter is written by acknowledged experts in their field. A detailed introduction to the physiology of pain by Mark Johnson has been included to enable readers to update and refresh their memories on a topic last encountered in training. Much has changed in this area in the past few years. Thereafter, chapters on skin trauma, pain at dressing change, pain assessment, and, skin allergy provide up-to-date and authoritative reviews of our current knowledge.

The quality of life aspects are addressed in a chapter on leg ulcer pain by Douglas. This is a particularly exciting topic as, until very recently, it was not generally recognised that leg ulcer patients were subject to significant pain. This theme is developed by Price in her chapter on the psychological aspects of pain. This is something for all practitioners involved in wound care to be aware of.

The significance of wound pain in specific wound types, together with the medical management of pain, complement these chapters to provide what is likely to become a standard reference text in the area of pain and wound healing. This book provides, for the first time, a single source of reference for many of the complex component parts of this aspect of clinical practice. It will provide essential information and insight to the practicing clinician, and ensures that this aspect of patient care is considered as part of comprehensive patient management.

Richard White
Whitstone

June 2006

Section I: The nature of the problem

Chapter 1

The clinical significance of wound pain

Helen Hollinworth and Richard White

Wound-related pain has become both a professional and humanitarian concern, but practice will only change if all professionals actively engage in care strategies proven to minimise trauma and pain in wound care. The starting point is to understand the patients' experiences and the impact that wound-related pain has on their lives.

Wound pain needs to be as important to the practitioner as it is to the patient. The experience of pain in patients with wounds will impact on clinical outcomes.

Pain produces physiological stress which can adversely affect healing (Kiecolt-Glaser *et al*, 1995; Broadbent *et al*, 2003; McGuire *et al*, 2006); in addition, it increases blood pressure and levels of cortisol 'stress hormone'. This latter phenomenon may non-specifically impair the inflammatory response in normal wound healing (Broadbent *et al*, 2003).

It is necessary to look at the aetiology of wound-related pain, when it occurs, associated procedures, and, the impact of pain on the clinical outcomes. Other chapters in this book will focus in detail on dressings and pain, assessment of pain at dressing change, and, skin trauma. This chapter considers how and when pain impacts on clinical outcomes.

Pain is described as having three major components:

❖ *Perceptive:* how much it hurts, eg. the physical sensation of having a wound.
❖ *Reactive:* the psychological aspect (*Chapter 9*) relates to the feelings of anxiety, depression and anger which may exacerbate

the patient's pain response. Pain catastrophising has been shown to be positively related to pain intensity and higher levels of affective distress and depressive symptoms in patients with chronic wounds (Roth *et al*, 2004).

❖ *Cognitive:* the attitudes and beliefs about pain.

The factors that give rise to wound pain have been defined (Hollinworth, 2000; Ryan *et al*, 2003; *Table 1.1*). Relating pain to various wounds types, it is possible to illustrate how pain impacts on clinical outcomes.

Table 1.1: Factors that may result in wound pain
• Trauma during dressing change
• Products used
• Skin excoriation
• Infection
• Lack of empathy
• Poor bandaging technique

Hollinworth, 2000

Wound pain: chronic wounds

Venous and arterial leg ulcers are often very painful (Mangwendeza, 2002; Ryan *et al*, 2003). The clinical factors contributing to this are numerous (*Table 2.1*). Ulcer pain can reduce patient quality of life (Heinen *et al*, 2004; Hareendran *et al*, 2005; Iglesias *et al*, 2005), particularly if not managed appropriately (Charles, 2002; Heinen *et al*, 2004), but this is not always the case (McMullen, 2004). The implementation of care models has been shown to improve clinical outcomes by reducing levels of pain and ulcer healing (Freedman *et al*, 2003; Charles, 2004; Edwards *et al*, 2005). Furthermore, by addressing the patient's pain, concordance with treatment can often be improved (Briggs, 2005).

Table 1.2: Clinical factors contributing to venous leg ulcer pain
• Oedema
• Onset of arterial disease
• Livedoid vasculitis, or atrophie blanche
• Dermatitis: acute phase — itching, redness, exudation
• Lipodermatosclerosis
• Compression
• Limb elevation

Mangwendeza, 2002

Wound pain: acute wounds

Much has been published on the clinical effects of post-operative pain on the healing response and patient quality of life (Shipton and Tait, 2005; Van Den Kerkhof _et al_, 2006). The Royal College of Surgeons (RCS) of England has stated in a report on pain after surgery that, 'treatment of pain after surgery is central to the care of post-operative patients. Failure to relieve pain is morally and ethically unacceptable' (RCS, 1990). However, since this report was issued there has been no audit or follow-up to monitor practice.

Dressing change procedures

Pain may arise through the traumatic removal of adherent dressings (_Chapter 4_). This can have numerous effects: it can lead to trauma of the surrounding skin and the wound bed, and such trauma will increase the time to healing (Hollinworth, 2005a) and involve extra time and materials. It is also possible that the trauma leads to infection, with a consequent increase in costs and morbidity.

Perhaps it has never occurred to us that the methods used to cleanse wounds or remove dressings could give rise to unnecessary pain for our patients. Our patients may grimace but they rarely say anything. Alternatively, pain may be recognised, but not treated. Evidence-based practice has become the mantra of modern health care, but even when clinical guidelines are available (European Wound Management Association [EWMA], 2002; World Union of Wound Healing Societies [WUWHS], 2004; Independent Advisory Group, 2004), practice frequently remains unchanged (Tendra Academy Expert Forum, 2006). Financial constraints and organisational change impact on the time available for wound care activities, and the type of relationship practitioners can develop with their patients, and yet assessment and psychological support are critical components of person-centred care. Entrenched traditional practices and our reluctance to challenge professional colleagues perceived as being more powerful, serve to compound our feelings of disempowerment. This is important because disempowered practitioners are unlikely to empower patients who have wounds, or their families. Counter to this perspective, is recognition that every practitioner is accountable for their own professional practice, and poor practice increasingly results in litigation (Dimond, 2003; Dimond, 2005). This serves to emphasise that forcefully removing dressings that have adhered to the wound bed, or adhesive products that cause tissue trauma on removal, can be considered inhumane (Human Rights Act, 1998). It is imperative that all healthcare professionals critically evaluate current practice.

In clinical practice, much of the pain and tissue trauma patients experience during wound care procedures can be reduced, often considerably. Inadequate holistic assessment and management of pain, inappropriate wound management strategies, and practitioners who distance themselves from patients' experiences, are just some of the many causes of wound-related pain (Hollinworth, 2005a). Exploring these causes in more detail implicates traditional dressings, some modern dressings, wound debridement, infection, underlying aetiology (eg. leg ulcers, burns and scalds), and an insensitive approach or rough handling of the patient's limb or wound. Dressing removal has been repeatedly identified as the time when patients experience the most wound pain and tissue trauma (Moffatt *et al*, 2002; Bethell, 2003; Jones and San Miguel, 2006). However, there are also many practical strategies that can be readily incorporated into clinical practice to address these issues. Assessment provides a logical starting point (Hollinworth, 2005b), but understanding the patient's experience is critical.

Understanding the patient's experience

Professional practice exposes a host of circumstances when patients experience painful wounds, but sometimes practitioners fail to understand the impact of a painful wound and living with pain on a day-to-day basis has on an individual. Pain assessment is particularly challenging in cognitively-impaired patients (Holen *et al*, 2005). For all patients, in all age groups, there is a professional tension in practice only focused on a wound care procedure, without acknowledging the patient as a person (Hollinworth, 2005a). Wound care requires a paradigm shift towards person-centred care; it is no longer acceptable that this is just an approach to which professionals aspire. Person-centred care must embrace psychological aspects of having a wound, experiences which may be compounded by anxiety, fear, and previous interventions that were painful. Unless we actively engage with our patients and assess the causes and type of their pain, the care that patients receive could be compromised. Sometimes patients have ongoing, background pain due to disease processes, such as arthritis or peripheral vascular disease (PVD), which may be present even at rest (WUWHS, 2004). Maintaining a gentle and sensitive approach when caring for patients, using thoughtful positioning of painful limbs, speaking on behalf of the patient if colleagues are rough in their approach, and limiting wound exposure time are all practical strategies to enhance care. Patients with venous leg ulceration repeatedly describe pain as being the overwhelming feature impacting on their lives (Chase *et al*, 1997; Douglas, 2001), and pain and powerlessness encapsulated the experiences of patients with peripheral vascular disease (Gibson and Kenrick, 1998). The physical and emotional suffering of people with chronic or malodorous wounds are recurring themes in the literature that mirror many practitioners concerns (Neil and Munjas, 2000; Hack, 2003; Goode, 2004). These clinical issues underline the importance of understanding the physiology and psychological effects of pain. It is also important to understand why dressing changes can be such painful procedures for our patients.

Dressings that have adhered to the wound bed

A common cause of trauma and wound pain is adhered dressings. Removal of dressings that have adhered or become stuck to the wound bed frequently traumatises the wound, causing significant pain for the patient, and further extends healing by reverting the wound back to the inflammatory stage each time the dressing is changed. Traditional products, gauze and paraffin tulle (eg. Jelonet™, Smith & Nephew), have been repeatedly shown to adhere to the wound bed in this way, and, if left *in situ*, granulation tissue grows into the product mesh, exacerbating problems of adherence, with wound pain and trauma on removal (Hollinworth and Collier, 2000; Bethell, 2003; Jones and San Miguel, 2006). It is a professional concern that this practice still persists. Use of these products is still seen clinically in the management of donor sites, dressing the nail bed following toe-nail removal, and packing of some cavity wounds, an example being pilonidal sinus cavity wounds. It would appear that insufficient consideration is given to the patient's experience of pain and the detrimental effect on healing, largely on the basis of ritualistic practice and initial unit cost. However, low unit cost needs to be balanced against the more expensive costs of nursing time and dressing packs for repeated dressing changes, analgesia costs, potential increased risks of infection, and patient inconvenience. The cosmetic result also needs to be considered. In practice, saline-soaked gauze requires at least 4-hourly dressing changes to avoid adherence, and daily dressing changes for paraffin gauze. Problems of adherence to the wound bed also occur with modern products, such as so-called 'low-adherent' products, because of the viscous, 'glue-like' nature of drying exudate (Rogers *et al*, 1999). Where there is minimal exudate, some dressings are able to handle the fluid by having a 'breathable' outer covering, which functions in a similar way to the stratum corneum. This 'breathability' in a dressing is described as the moisture vapour transpiration rate (MVTR). The higher the dressing MVTR, the greater the dressing's capacity to allow fluid to evaporate (Bolton *et al*, 2000). This method of managing fluid is only suitable for low amounts of exudate, but is often used as part of a combined approach.

When adherence occurs, practitioners often resort to soaking with water or normal saline in an effort to ease removal. Unfortunately, this strategy is rarely effective (Hollinworth and Collier, 2000), and is time-consuming and stressful for both patient and practitioner. Having identified problems of adherence, this must be documented, and appropriate changes made to future care (Hollinworth, 2005b).

Case study

Some of the clinical issues explored in this introductory chapter are illustrated by the following example drawn from professional practice. Practitioners working in an intermediate care setting, recognised that they were having difficulty in healing the sacral pressure ulcer of a lady in her early seventies (despite appropriate pressure-relieving equipment) and, therefore, sought advice.

Observation of care exposed several clinical issues:

* Moving the patient onto her side to facilitate the dressing change required considerable effort by the carers, and even then access to the sacral area was limited. This resulted in carers

pulling at sacral tissues in their efforts to remove the adhesive product. The outcome was considerable tissue trauma to the skin around the ulcer.

❖ The patient displayed facial expressions of discomfort during movement, and called out in pain during dressing removal. There had been no prior assessment of pain, and the approach to care lacked sensitivity.

❖ Exudate seeping onto peri-wound tissue had resulted in macerated wound margins, but no attempts to address this increased risk of tissue trauma were incorporated into the care plan.

❖ Pressurised normal saline from a canister was used for cleansing the wound. The unpleasant sensation from the saline jet clearly caused further pain for the patient; this was compounded by gauze being drawn across the wound on the premise of drying the area.

These common clinical issues are a professional concern. However, framed by subsequent chapters, such examples can serve as a springboard for enhanced patient-centred wound care in the future.

Adhesive products and tapes causing tissue trauma on removal

Another clinical issue is the tissue trauma caused by adhesive dressings and tapes used to secure products in place (*Figure 1.1*). The strength of the adhesive on the product has implications for the extent of tissue trauma, or stripping of the epidermis from around the wound, as the dressing or tape is removed (Dykes *et al*, 2001; Zillmer *et al*, 2006). As with adhered dressings, soaking to aid removal has limited effect, as the adhesive bond resists the effects of solutions, such as water or normal saline in the majority of cases (Hollinworth and Collier, 2000). Removing products with aggressive adhesives can readily cause blisters when the epidermis is pulled away from the dermis, even with healthy skin. The problem is exacerbated on delicate fragile skin, a common condition in the elderly person and young children. The effects of prolonged topical and systemic steroid therapy, or skin conditions such as epidermolysis bullosa (EB), compound the situation. Tissue trauma caused by adhesives may occur with post-operative dressings, tapes used to secure non-adhesive dressings in place, and the many different dressings that incorporate an adhesive either over their whole surface, or around a central dressing. Again, it is important to assess for this type of tissue trauma as products are removed, and instigate strategies that minimise the problem. Tissue trauma caused by removing adhesive products, or tapes, can frequently extend the size of the wound or ulcer, exacerbate existing wound pain, and further delay healing. The emotional impact on the patient also needs to be considered.

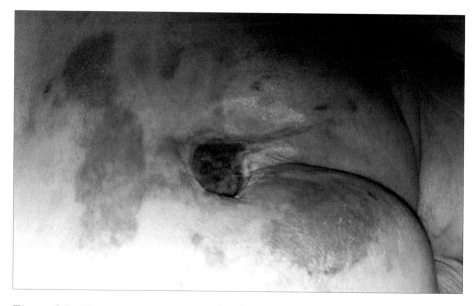

Figure 1.1: Tissue trauma as a result of removing adherent products

Linked to the use of adhesives is the issue of allergic contact sensitivity (Farm, 1998). Patients who have been exposed to a range of different wound management products over a period of time, for example, venous leg ulcer patients, readily develop contact sensitivities (Tavadia *et al*, 2003; see *Chapter 6*). Adhesives have frequently been implicated (Fraki *et al*, 1979; Ratcliffe, 2001). This is important clinically, as the risk of contact sensitivity impacts on product choice, patient concordance with planned care, and may heighten wound-related pain.

Tissue excoriation due to wound exudate

A clinical issue that frequently exacerbates a wound or ulcer is the problem of tissue excoriation due to wound exudate. Products that inadequately manage the amount of exudate produced by a wound, or fail to adequately control the moisture balance at the wound/dressing interface, cause excoriation, irritant dermatitis, and/or maceration of peri-wound tissues (Cutting and White, 2002a). Wound exudate has been described as a 'corrosive' biological fluid (Bishop *et al*, 2003) and, as such, should be regarded as a wounding agent in its own right (Chen, 1996). This tissue trauma can cause considerable discomfort for the patient, and the size of the wound may extend, which further delays healing. Chronic wound exudate contains high concentrations of proteolytic enzymes that readily cause tissue and cellular damage to the delicate tissue around the margins of wounds (Moore, 2003). Chronic wound fluid in prolonged contact with peri-wound tissues can precipitate an eczematous-type reaction, and can cause maceration of these tissues (Cutting and White, 2002b). Excess skin wetness, or maceration, is indicated by a white coloration of peri-wound tissues, and renders the tissue prone to trauma and consequent wound enlargement (White and Cutting, 2003). Some practitioners attempt to protect the tissues with a range of barrier creams or moisturisers, although only a few have supporting clinical evidence (Cameron *et al*, 2005). It is important to assess for tissue excoriation, or maceration of peri-wound tissues, and explore the wide range of options that can make a real difference to the patient's care and quality of life. However, maceration is a problem best avoided as 'recovery' is very difficult to achieve (Cutting and White, 2002b).

Wound cleansing issues

It is hard to understand why patients are still subjected to wound cleansing strategies that exacerbate their existing pain, and often cause further trauma to delicate healing tissues. The first step is to consider why the wound or ulcer is being cleansed, because many practitioners inextricably link wound dressing changes with wound cleansing. Wounds do not routinely require cleansing. Wiping across the wound or ulcer bed with gauze readily traumatises fragile granulation tissue, and, on virtually every occasion, it is a painful, unpleasant experience for the patient. Imagine if you had an open wound and someone dragged, sometimes repeatedly, pieces of gauze across it. Alternatively, imagine that you have a leg ulcer that has been immersed in water, but then the person caring for you not only washes your leg, but also rubs up and down on the ulcer itself. These common practices should not continue.

If product residues require removal from the wound bed or peri-wound skin, then gentle irrigation with a warm, isotonic solution can be used, although critical evaluation of product choice may be necessary. The ideal irrigation technique is still undecided, despite 30 years of research (Chatterjee, 2005). In traumatic wounds, initial irrigation with an antiseptic solution may be appropriate, but all professionals need to be aware of the intense stinging associated with antiseptics, and manage the patient's pain accordingly. High-pressure irrigation for traumatic injuries should only be used in a controlled environment, with personal protective equipment worn due to 'splash back', and adequate pain control for the patient. If a foreign body such as gravel is embedded in a superficial trauma wound, a hydrocolloid dressing can aid removal after 24/48 hours in a relatively pain-free manner. Irrigating any wound is unlikely to remove adherent slough, or significantly reduce the microbial load of the wound for any clinically-meaningful length of time. The systematic approaches to wound assessment and management, such as 'Wound Bed Preparation/TIME', and 'Applied Wound Management' (AWM) embrace alternative approaches to these issues (Dowsett and Newton, 2005; Gray et al, 2005).

Conclusion

There is now abundant evidence that pain can have both a physical and emotional impact on the patient. In the process of wound management, pain is often related to the quality of care provided. Outdated practices must be challenged. Wound pain and tissue trauma should not be trivialised or treated without due consideration; we now have effective guidelines and products for the 'modern' management of wounds in a relatively pain-free and atraumatic way.

References

Beldon P (2006) Avoiding allergic contact dermatitis in patients with venous leg ulcers. *Br J Community Nurs* **11**(3): S6–S12

Bethell E (2003) Why gauze dressings should not be the first choice to manage most acute surgical cavity wounds. *J Wound Care* **12**(6): 237–9

Bishop S, Walker M, Rogers A, Chen W (2003) The importance of moisture balance at the wound-dressing interface. *J Wound Care* **12**(4): 125–8

Bolton LL, Monte K, Pione LA (2000) Moisture and healing: beyond the jargon. *Ostomy/Wound Management* **46**(suppl 1A): 51S–62S

Briggs SL (2005) Leg ulcer management: how addressing a patient's pain can improve concordance. *Prof Nurs* **20**(6): 39–41

Broadbent E, Petrie KJ, Alley PG, Booth RJ (2003) Psychological stress impairs early wound repair following surgery. *Psychosom Med* **65**(5): 865–9

Cameron J, Hofman D, Wilson J, Cherry G (2005) Comparison of two peri-wound skin protectants in venous leg ulcers: a randomised controlled trial. *J Wound Care* **14**(5): 233–6

Charles H (2002) Venous leg ulcer pain and its characteristics. *J Tissue Viability* **12**(4): 154–8

Charles H (2004) Does leg ulcer treatment improve patients' quality of life. *J Wound Care* **13**(6): 209–13

Chase SK, Melloni M, Savage A (1997) A forever healing: the lived experience of venous ulcer disease. *J Vascular Nurs* **15**(2): 73–8

Chatterjee J (2005) A critical review of irrigation techniques in acute wounds. *Int Wound J* **2**(3): 258–65

Chen J (1996) In: Aquacel Hydrofiber® dressing: the next step in wound dressing technology. Monograph, ConvaTec UK

Cutting KF, White RJ (2002a) Maceration of the skin 1: the nature and causes of skin maceration. *J Wound Care* **11**(7): 275–8

Cutting KF, White RJ (2002b) Avoidance and management of peri-wound skin maceration. *Prof Nurs* **18**(1): 33–6

Dimond B (2003) Legal concerns in tissue viability and wound healing. *Nurs Standard* **17**(23): 70–6

Dimond B (2005) Litigation and pressure ulcers. In: Glover D, ed. *Science of Surfaces*. Hill Rom in association with Journal of Wound Care, January

Douglas V (2001) Living with a chronic leg ulcer: an insight into patients' experiences and feelings. *J Wound Care* **10**(9): 355–60

Dowsett C, Newton H. (2005) Wound bed preparation: TIME in practice. *Wounds UK* **1**(3): 58–70

Dykes P, Heggie R, Hill S (2001) Effects of adhesive dressings on the stratum corneum of the skin. *J Wound Care* **10**(2): 7–10

Edwards H, Courtney M, Finlayson K *et al* (2005) Chronic venous leg ulcers: effect of a community nursing intervention on pain and healing. *Nurs Standard* **19**(52): 47–54

European Wound Management Association (EWMA) (2002) *Position Document: Pain at wound dressing changes*. Medical Education Partnership Ltd, London

Farm G (1998) Contact allergy to colophony. *Acta Derm Venereol* (Stockh) **201**: 1–42

Fraki JE, Peltonen L, Hopsu-Havu VK (1979) Allergy to various components of topical preparations in stasis dermatitis and leg ulcer. *Contact Derm* **5**(2): 97–100

Freedman G, Cean C, Duron V *et al* (2003) Pathogensis and treatment of pain in patients with chronic wounds. *Surg Technol Int* **11**: 168–79

Gibson J, Kenrick M (1998) Pain and powerlessness: the experience of living with peripheral vascular disease. *J Adv Nurs* **27**: 737–45

Goode M (2004) Psychological needs of patients when dressing a fungating wound: a literature review. *J Wound Care* **13**(9): 380–2

Gray DG, White RJ, Cooper P, Kingsley AR (2005) Understanding Applied Wound Management. *Wounds UK* **1**(1): 62–70

Hack A (2003) Malodorous wounds — taking the patient's perspective into account. *J Wound Care* **12**(8): 319–21

Hareendran A, Bradbury A, Budd J *et al* (2005) Measuring the impact of venous leg ulcers on quality of life. *J Wound Care* **14**(2): 53–7

Heinen MM, van Achterberg T, op Reimer WS *et al* (2004) Venous leg ulcer patients: a review of the literature on lifestyle and pain-related interventions. *J Clin Nurs* **13**(3): 355–66

Holen J C, Saltvedt I, Fayers P M, Bjornnes M *et al* (2005) The Norwegian Doloplus-2, a tool for behavioural pain assessment: translation and pilot validation in nursing home patients with cognitive impairment. *Palliat Med* **19**(5): 411–17

Hollinworth H (2005a) The management of patients' pain in wound care, *Nurs Standard* **20**(7): 65–73

Hollinworth H (2005b) Pain at wound dressing-related procedures: a template for assessment. Available online at: www.worldwidewounds. com/2005/august/Hollinworth/Framework-Assessing-Pain-Wound-Dressing-Related.html (accessed 3 April, 2006)

Hollinworth H, Collier M (2000) Nurses' views about pain and trauma at dressing changes: results of a national survey. *J Wound Care* 9(8): 369–73

Human Rights Act (1998) Article 3. The Stationery Office, London

Iglesias CP, Birks Y, Nelson EA *et al* (2005) Quality of life of people with venous leg ulcers: a comparison of the discriminative and responsive characteristics of two generic and disease specific instruments. *Qual Life Res* 14(7): 1705–18

Independent Advisory Group (2004) *Best practice statement: Minimising trauma and pain in wound management.* Wounds UK, Aberdeen. Available online at: www.wounds-uk.com

Jones A, San Miguel L (2006) Are modern wound dressings a clinical and cost-effective alternative to gauze? *J Wound Care* 15(2): 65–9

Kiecolt-Glaser JK, Marucha PT, Malarkey WB *et al* (1995) Slowing of wound healing by psychological stress. *Lancet* 346(8984): 1194–6

McGuire L, Heffner K, Glaser R *et al* (2006) Pain and wound healing in surgical patients. *Ann Behav Med* 31(2): 165–72

McMullen M (2004) The relationship between pain and leg ulcers: a critical review. *Br J Nurs* 13(19): S30–S36

Mangwendeza A (2002) Pain in venous leg ulceration: aetiology and management. *Br J Nurs* 11(19): 1237–42

Moffatt C, Franks P, Hollinworth H (2002) Understanding wound pain and trauma: an international perspective. In: European Wound Management Association *Pain at Wound Dressing Changes: Position Document.* Medical Education Partnership, London.

Moore K (2003) Compromised wound healing: a scientific approach to healing. *Br J Community Nurs* 8(6): 274–8

Neil J, Munjas B (2000) Living with a chronic wound: the voices of sufferers. *Ostomy/Wound Management* 46(5): 28–38

Ratcliffe J (2001) Reactions to topical medicaments and wound care products. *NT Plus* 97(35): 59–62

Rogers AA, Walmsley RS, Rippon MG, Bowler PG (1999) Adsorption of serum-derived proteins by primary dressings: implications for dressing adhesion to wounds. *J Wound Care* 8(8): 403–6

Roth RS, Lowery JC, Hamill JB (2004) Assessing persistent pain and its relation to affective distress, depressive symptoms, and pain catastrophizing in patients with chronic wounds: a pilot study. *Am J Phys Med Rehab* 83(11): 827–34

Royal College of Surgeons (1990) Royal College of Surgeons of England. Commission on the provision of surgical services: Report of the working party on pain after surgery. RCS, London

Ryan S, Eager C, Sibbald RG (2003) Venous leg ulcer pain. *Ostomy/Wound Management* **49**(4): Suppl 16–23

Shipton EA, Tait B (2005) Flagging the pain: preventing the burden of chronic pain by identifying and treating the risk factors in acute pain. *Eur J Anaesthesiol* **22**(6): 405–12

Tavadia S, Bianchi J, Dawe RS *et al* (2003) Allergic contact dermatitis in venous leg ulcer patients. *Contact Derm* **48**(5): 261–5

Tendra Academy Expert Forum (2006) *Issues in wound care: implementing best practice to minimise trauma and pain.* Mölnlycke Health Care, Dunstable

Van Den Kerkhof EG, Hopman WM, Towheed T *et al* (2006) Pain, health-related quality of life and health care utilization: a pilot study. *Pain Res Management* **11**(1): 41–7

White RJ, Cutting KF (2003) Interventions to avoid maceration of the skin and wound bed. *Br J Nurs* **12**(20): 1186–1201

World Union of Wound Healing Societies (2004) *Principles of Best Practice: Minimising pain at wound dressing-related procedures. A consensus document.* Available online at: www.wuwhs.org/pdf/consensus_eng.pdf

Zillmer R, Karlsmark T, Ágren MS, Gottrup F (2006) Biophysical effects of repetitive removal of adhesive dressings on the skin surrounding ulcers. *J Wound Care* **15**(5): 1–5

CHAPTER 2

PHYSIOLOGY OF PAIN

Mark Johnson

Wound pain is a problem

The European Wound Management Association (EWMA) Position Document acknowledges that pain is a major issue for patients with wounds, and that inadequate treatment of wound pain has been consistently reported (European Wound Management Association Position Document, 2002). Wound pain may be associated with underlying pathology of the wound and/or wound management, such as debridement or dressing changes (Krasner, 1995). An international survey of 11 countries which formed part of the EWMA document, found that patients experience greatest pain during dressing change, and that practitioners rank prevention of pain and wound trauma as the most desired characteristic at a dressing change (Moffatt *et al*, 2002). Interestingly however, practitioners from only 2 of 11 countries rated giving analgesia as the most important factor before dressing changes (of 8 possible options).

Misguided beliefs

Practitioners often give wound pain management a low priority because they are preoccupied with treating visible pathology. Insufficient prescribing of analgesia also results from inappropriate pain assessment and the belief that pain is harmless and an unavoidable consequence of having a wound, which is not the case. Some practitioners have misguided fears of addiction and/or respiratory depression associated with opioid analgesics (Ready and Edwards, 1992; Cousins and Power 1999).

Misguided beliefs often result from insufficient knowledge about the physiology of pain. Pain is a psychological state that produces a state of physiological stress, and this is detrimental to health and will slow the healing process. Pain increases blood pressure, alters blood gases, delays gastric emptying, causes urinary retention, and increases levels of 'stress hormones' such as cortisol (*Figure 2.1*).

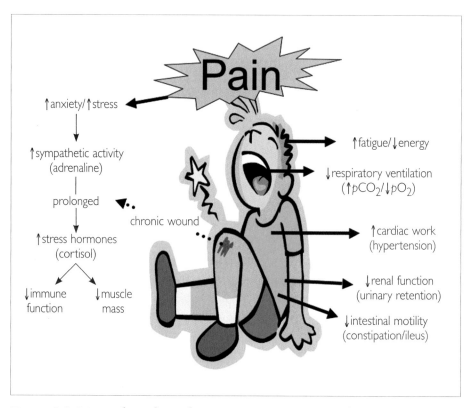

Figure 2.1: Many physiological responses to pain are mediated through the sympathetic division of the autonomic nervous system

Unfortunately, learning about the physiology of pain is often painful in itself because too much attention is given to its physiological components. Despite what physiologists may have you believe, practitioners do not need to know the names of all of the molecule substrates that may be involved in pain processing. It is far more important for practitioners to have a working knowledge of the physiological concepts that underpin the types of pain seen in the clinical setting. The purpose of this chapter is to overview the physiological concepts that help in our understanding of pain.

What is pain?

Defining pain

In clinical practice, 'Pain is what the patient says it is' (McCaffery, 1983) and, therefore, related to the person's ability to articulate what they are experiencing. Leg ulceration and superficial burns have been reported to be the most painful wounds with pressure ulcers, cuts, abrasions, and fungating wounds less painful (Moffatt *et al*, 2002). However, 'most painful' and 'less painful' are general terms and give little insight to the exact nature of a patient's experience. Patients usually use the term 'pain' in conjunction with adjectives about of the intensity of the pain, the quality of the pain, the extent of the pain, or how bothersome the pain is. These adjectives are crucial in establishing the nature of a patient's pain and are influenced by many factors including type of injury, culture, environment, and individual circumstance (Melzack, 1975; Melzack and Katz, 1999).

The International Association for the Study of Pain (IASP) defines pain as:

> *... an unpleasant sensory and emotional experience associated with actual or potential tissue damage, or described in terms of such damage.*

(Merskey and Bogduk, 1994)

This working definition demonstrates that pain is a psychological state and, therefore, a personal experience and always subjective.

The nociceptive system

The body's neural system dedicated to detecting actual or potential tissue damage (ie. noxious stimuli) is called the nociceptive system and consists of:

* *Nociceptors:* Sensory receptor cells preferentially sensitive to noxious stimuli or to stimuli which would become noxious if prolonged (Merskey and Bogduk, 1994).
* *Transmission pathways:* Neural pathways sending nerve impulses from nociceptors to, and within, the central nervous system.
* *Processing areas (perception):* Neural areas in the brain which process incoming impulses to generate an awareness of the noxious stimulus via the sensation of pain (*Figure 2.2*).

However, the IASP definition avoids linking all pain to the presence of tissue damage because the relationship between pain and injury is sometimes very variable.

Pain is difficult to predict

Injury is not always a good predictor of pain, as demonstrated in the following examples:

* an injury may occur without pain, as seen in neuropathic foot ulcers where the reduced sensibility leads to a chronic wound
* an injury may generate pain that is out of proportion to the extent of tissue damage, as seen when a sliver of metal embeds under a finger nail producing excruciating pain
* an injury may have healed yet pain persists, as seen in post-amputation stump pain
* an injury may amplify the intensity of subsequent stimuli, as seen during wound dressings
* an injury may generate pain at a different body location, as seen in referred pain down the arm during a myocardial infarction.

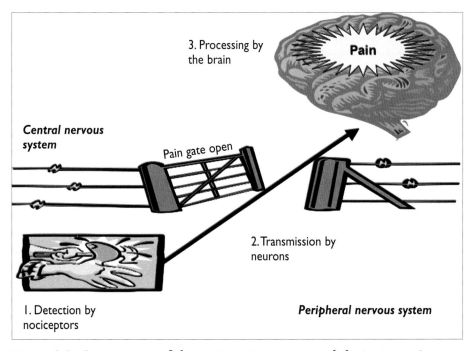

Figure 2.2: Components of the nociceptive system and the 'pain gate'. Activity in the nociceptive neurons opens the 'pain gate' so that impulses can reach higher levels of the brain where they are processed to create a sensation of pain

Pain is a multidimensional experience

Pain consists of sensory-discriminative, affective-motivational, and cognitive-evaluative dimensions (Melzack and Katz, 1999; *Figure 2.3*).

* *Sensory-discriminative dimensions* relate to the intensity, location, and quality of the pain, and are sub-served by the nociceptive system and its association with the somatosensory cortex.
* *Affective-motivational dimensions* relate to emotional aspects of pain and are sub-served by the nociceptive system and its association with the reticular and limbic systems (insula cortex and cingulate gyrus).
* *Cognitive-evaluative dimensions* relate to thoughts and meanings of pain and are sub-served by the nociceptive system and its association with the frontal lobe of the cerebral cortex.

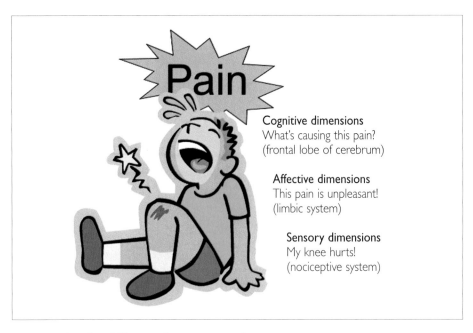

Figure 2.3: The different dimensions of pain

Each dimension of the pain experience must be addressed during treatment and, therefore, a multidisciplinary pain management approach is necessary. Pain of known cause and limited duration, such as minor cuts and abrasions, have modest contributions from affective and cognitive dimensions because the patient expects the pain to disappear as the injury heals. Pain that persists, such as a chronic leg ulcer pain, may have substantial contributions from affective and cognitive dimensions, because the patient does not understand why the wound does not heal.

Pain is a dynamic entity

Pain is a dynamic phenomenon that will fluctuate in quality, intensity, and location over time (ie. seconds, minutes, hours, days, months and years). Wound pain may exist when the patient is resting and in the absence of external stimuli (ie. background pain). Background pain may persist throughout the day (ie. static or continuous), or it may be intermittent (episodic). Intermittent pain may be erratic or it may occur in waves and patterns (*Figure 2.4*). There may be a background pain which flares up intermittently from time to time. Wounds are often sensitive to provoking stimuli as occurs during dressing changes or debridement. These provoking stimuli produce particularly intense and distressing pain, which is substantially amplified and out of proportion to the intensity of provoking stimulus.

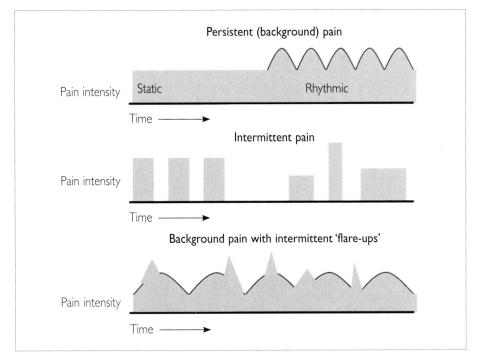

Figure 2.4: Patterns of pain

The nociceptive system can alter its sensitivity

The nociceptive system operates in various states of sensitivity as characterised in *Table 2.1* (Woolf, 1987; Woolf, 1994; Woolf and Salter, 2000).

This is evident if you consider progress of a typical 'household injury', such as a graze or a burn to the skin (*Figure 2.5*).

Table 2.1: The characteristics of normal, suppressed and sensitised pain (adapted from Doubell et al, 1999)

Nociceptive system state	Nociceptive transmission	Peripheral tissue	Afferent input	Sensation	Clinical correlate
Normal (control)	Normal	Healthy	Non-noxious Noxious	No pain Pain	Transient pain
Sensitised	Amplified due to increased excitation or reduced inhibition	Injured	Non-noxious Noxious	Pain (allodynia) Exaggerated pain (hyperalgesia)	Nociceptive and/or neuropathic pain
Persistently sensitised and/or reorganised	May be amplified or abnormal	May be healthy or injured	Non-noxious Noxious	Pain (allodynia) Exaggerated pain (hyperalgesia)	Persistent nociceptive and/or neuropathic pain
Suppressed	Diminished due to reduced excitation or increased inhibition	Healthy or injured	Non-noxious Noxious	No pain Reduced pain	Pain relief

Normal state

The nociceptive system operates in a 'normal state' in healthy individuals who do not have any appreciable tissue damage. In its normal state, the nociceptive system is primed to detect actual or potential tissue damage. When a noxious stimulus occurs, such as spillage of boiling water on to a hand, the nociceptive system will instigate a rapid reflex withdrawal of the body part from the source of the tissue damage. This often occurs before you experience pain (*Figure 2.6*).

A few seconds later, a sharp, intense, localised pain develops (termed first or fast pain) followed by a dull, aching, spreading pain (termed second or slow pain) which is sometimes accompanied by nausea. These two pain sensations result from direct activation of the nociceptive system and their intensity mirrors the intensity of the stimuli. They help us to remember to avoid the stimuli in the future (*Figure 2.6*).

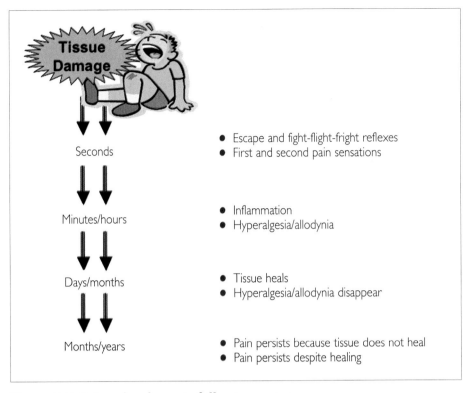

Figure 2.5: Pain-related events following an injury

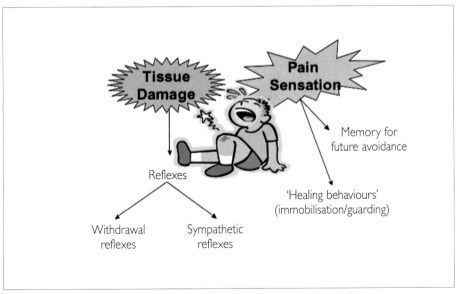

Figure 2.6: Immediate responses to injury when the nociceptive system is operating in its normal pre-injury state

Suppressed state

The nociceptive system can also operate in a 'suppressed state' whereby the intensity of pain is lower than expected. Pouring cold water over an injury or rubbing the skin close to the injury may provide immediate but short-term pain relief. Reducing pain in this way allows us to continue actions, such as completing an important sporting event, despite the presence of tissue damage. The nociceptive system can also be suppressed by mental distraction and motivational states.

Sensitised state

In healthy tissue, low intensity stimuli produce non-painful sensations, such as touch, hot, cold, and high intensity stimuli produce pain. However, in the presence of tissue damage, low intensity stimuli produce increased pain (allodynia), and high intensity stimuli produce exaggerated pain (hyperalgesia). For example, touching an open wound with your finger produces pain, instead of touch, and pricking an open wound with a needle produces excruciating pain that has a far higher intensity than would be expected for healthy tissue.

In damaged tissue, the nociceptive system operates in a 'sensitised state' to encourage behaviours that guard the injury from further damage and this will aid tissue healing. The sensitised state is recognised by pain in the absence of provoking stimuli (spontaneous pain), tenderness (allodynia), and exaggerated pain (hyperalgesia). Allodynia is, 'pain due to a stimulus which does not normally provoke pain' (Merskey and Bogduk, 1994). Hyperalgesia is, 'an increased response to a stimulus which is normally painful' (Merskey and Bogduk, 1994). Primary hyperalgesia occurs at the site of injury and secondary hyperalgesia occurs in the healthy tissue that surrounds the injury (Merskey and Bogduk, 1994).

Persistently sensitised state — dysfunctional

Normally, the nociceptive system returns to its normal pre-injury state when tissue heals and spontaneous pain, allodynia and hyperalgesia disappear. Sometimes the injury does not heal and the nociceptive system remains sensitised, as seen in some chronic wounds. Sometimes the injury heals but the nociceptive system remains sensitised, as seen when nerves have been injured. In these persistently sensitised states, the nociceptive system may well have developed its own pathophysiology and have become dysfunctional itself (Devor and Seltzer, 1999).

Categorising types of pain

Categorisation of pain is fraught with difficulty. Pain has been categorised according to: i) duration (eg. acute, chronic); ii) cause (eg. burn, pressure ulcer); iii) anatomical site (eg. back, headache); iv) system (eg. visceral, musculoskeletal); and v) physiological mechanism (eg. nociceptive, neuropathic), to name but a few. Often authors mix category systems in discussions and this has led to confusion in nomenclature and understanding. The most commonly used categorisation of pain in clinical practice is according to the duration of the pain as characterised in *Table 2.2*.

Transient pain (normal state)

Transient pain is 'pain of brief duration and little consequence....' (Melzack and Wall, 1988). It serves to initiate protective responses and to make us aware of stimuli that are damaging so that we can avoid them in the future (*Figure 2.6*, *Table 2.2*).

Acute pain (sensitised state)

Acute pain is 'pain of recent onset and probable limited duration. It usually has an identifiable temporal and causal relationship to injury and disease' (Ready and Edwards, 1992). Acute pain serves to aid tissue repair by making injured areas sensitive to provoking stimuli, as seen during wound dressing changes. Sensations of tenderness (allodynia) and exaggerated pain (hyperalgesia) are often present to promote behaviours that guard and/or immobilise the injured site (*Table 2.2*).

Chronic pain (persistently sensitised state — dysfunctional)

Chronic pain is '....pain lasting for long periods of time' (Ready and Edwards, 1992). Often, 'chronic pain commonly persists beyond the expected time of healing of an injury and frequently there may not be any clearly identifiable cause' (Ready and Edwards, 1992). However, pain may also persist because of ongoing tissue damage as seen in chronic wounds which fail to heal, or in degenerating disease such as arthritis or advanced cancer. Often, chronic pain serves no useful purpose and the nociceptive system itself may have become dysfunctional (*Table 2.2*).

Nociception — the normal pain state

Physiological responses to noxious stimuli

In healthy individuals a noxious stimulus generates a variety of physiological responses.

Withdrawal (somatic) reflexes

If you pick up something that is 'burning hot' you may well drop it before you experience a sensation of pain. This protective reflex, termed the withdrawal reflex, enables a rapid response to occur without us having to 'think about it'. The withdrawal reflex involves activation of tissue damage receptors (nociceptors), resulting in activity in afferent nociceptive neurons, interneurons in the spinal cord, efferent motor neurons and, ultimately, contraction and relaxation of opposing skeletal muscle groups (*Figure 2.7*).

Table 2.2: The characteristics of transient, acute and chronic pain

Characteristic	Transient pain	Acute pain	Chronic pain
Provoking stimulus	Noxious causing potential tissue damage	Noxious causing actual tissue damage	Persistent, ongoing tissue damage, or dysfunctional nociceptive system or unknown/other factors
Intensity and time course of pain sensation resulting from stimulus	Related to the severity of stimulus but usually short-lived and of little consequence if tissue damage is minimal	Related to the severity of stimulus and will diminish as tissue heals	May be predictable in the presence of ongoing disease or no relationship between pain and original injury (stimulus)
Status of tissue	Healthy	Damaged	May be healthy or damaged
Response to additional provoking stimuli	Normal Non-noxious stimuli produce non-noxious sensations Noxious stimuli produce pain	Amplified Non-noxious stimuli produce noxious sensations (allodynia) Noxious stimuli produce exaggerated pain (hyperalgesia)	Amplified Non-noxious stimuli produce noxious sensations (allodynia) Noxious stimuli produce exaggerated pain (hyperalgesia)
Physiological symptoms	Nociceptive system activated	Nociceptive system sensitised	Nociceptive system continuously activated and sensitised Nociceptive system dysfunctional and persistently sensitised
Function	Initiate escape responses to reduce extent of damage Memory of pain-evoking stimuli enables future avoidance	Initiate behaviours that guard/immobilise site of injury to prevent further tissue damage and to promote healing	Initiate behaviours that guard/immobilise site of injury to prevent further tissue damage and to promote healing Maladaptive — no clear purpose
Semantic correlates	Physiologic pain Nociceptive pain	Nociceptive pain Inflammatory pain	Persistent nociceptive/ inflammatory pain Neuropathic pain Pathophysiological pain

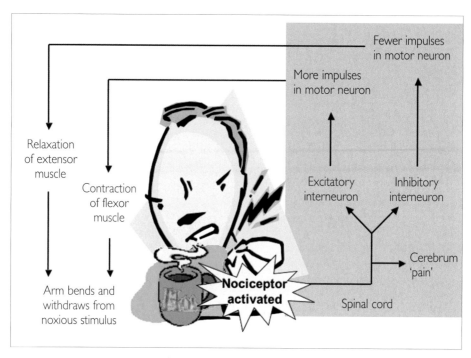

Figure 2.7: Components of the withdrawal reflex. Arrows indicate flow of neural information

The neural circuitry involved in the withdrawal reflex is likely to be involved in pains arising in skeletal muscle, such as nocturnal cramps and intermittent claudication associated with arterial disease. It is widely written that the tissue damage can cause persistent skeletal muscle contraction (spasm), leading to a pain-spasm-pain cycle whereby persistent skeletal muscle contraction activates muscle nociceptors and perpetuates a positive feedback loop (*Figure 2.8*). The idea that nociceptor activity causes muscle contraction which, in turn, generates further nociceptor activity causing further contraction has been challenged (Mense and Simons, 2001). Nevertheless, painful muscle spasms will compress blood vessels leading to skeletal muscle ischaemia. It is known that prolonged interruption of the blood supply to the skeletal muscles of resting limbs is not painful in itself. However, pain arises if ischaemic skeletal muscle begins to contract and will increase dramatically with increasing frequency, force, and duration of muscle contraction. These mechanisms are likely to contribute to muscle pains during nocturnal calf cramps seen with chronic venous insufficiency. These mechanisms also contribute to the deep-seated leg pain that occurs when patients with arterial disease walk a predictable distance (ie. intermittent claudication). These patients find that pain is relieved by a brief rest.

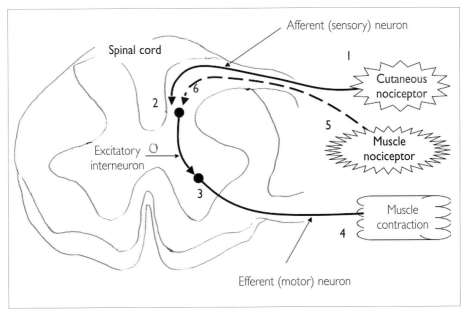

Figure 2.8: Motor reflexes contributing to pain. Activity in nociceptors [1] causes activation of interneurons [2] which, in turn, activate somatic efferent (motor) neurons [3]. Acetylcholine is released at the neuromuscular junction producing an intense and persistent muscle contraction [4] which is detected by muscle nociceptors [5]. The additional afferent information [dashed line] generates further muscle contraction via a positive feedback loop [6]. A positive feedback loop develops

Sympathetic (autonomic) reflexes

Noxious stimuli activate the sympathetic division of the autonomic nervous system (ANS) which releases adrenaline (epinephrine) and noradrenaline (norepinephrine). This causes a fight-flight-fright (stress-like) response and increased blood pressure, leading to hypertension, changes in pulmonary ventilation and alterations in blood gas concentrations, reductions in gastrointestinal motility and constipation, and reductions in bladder emptying and urinary retention (*Figure 2.1*).

In addition, noxious stimuli cause vasoconstriction in peripheral tissue leading to ischaemia, delayed tissue healing and enhanced nociceptor activity. The release of noradrenaline by sympathetic efferents at the site of tissue damage can sensitise nociceptors with the resultant increase in nociceptor activity forming positive feedback loops which exacerbate pain (*Figure 2.9*). Persistent pain will cause persistent sympathetic activity and an increase in the amount of circulating cortisol, thyroid hormones, and human growth hormone. Cortisol causes muscle wasting, suppression of the immune system, and possible gastrointestinal tract ulceration (Baron and Janig, 2004).

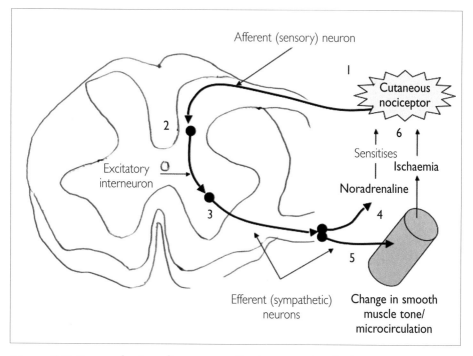

Figure 2.9: Sympathetic reflexes contributing to pain. Activity in nociceptors [1] causes activation of interneurons [2] and pre-ganglionic [3] and post-ganglionic sympathetic neurons. These sympathetic efferents release noradrenaline that sensitises cutaneous nociceptors [4] and causes vasoconstriction in peripheral tissue leading to ischaemia [5], resulting in more activity in nociceptors [6]. A positive feedback loop forms

Clearly, the plethora of reflex-induced physiological changes that occur as a result of nociceptor activity are complex and often additive. It is crucial that patients receive pain-relieving interventions to reduce their detrimental impact.

Psychological responses to noxious stimuli — the sensation of pain

In healthy individuals, a noxious stimulus may become a painful sensation through the processes of transduction, transmission, and perception (*Figures 2.2* and *2.10*).

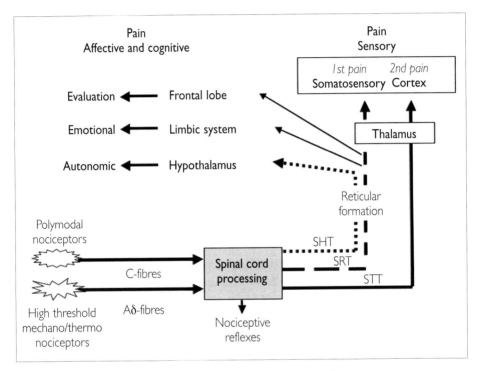

Figure 2.10: Nociceptor pathways and their relationship to sensory, affective and cognitive dimensions of pain. SRT = spinoreticular tract; STT = spinothalamic tract; SHT = spinohypothalamic tract

Transduction

Noxious, or tissue damaging stimuli are detected and converted into nerve impulses by nociceptors in a process called transduction. Nociceptors are, '[sensory] receptor(s) preferentially sensitive to a noxious stimulus or to a stimulus which would become noxious if prolonged' (Merskey and Bogduk, 1994). Nociceptors are 'tissue damage detectors', not 'pain detectors', because the sensation of pain is produced by the brain, not by the receptors. Nociceptors are free nerve endings that respond to high intensity thermal and mechanical stimuli and to chemicals produced by the body following injury (*Figure 2.11*) (Raja *et al*, 1999; Basbaum, 2004; Drew and Wood, 2004; Koltzenburg, 2004).

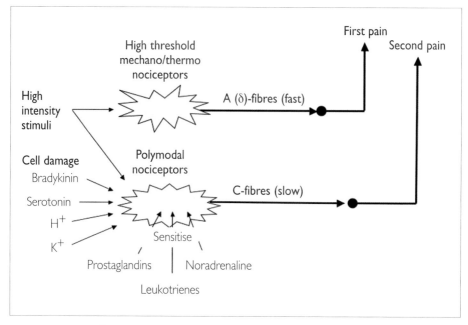

Figure 2.11: A-fibre and C-fibre nociceptors. C-fibre nociceptors are directly activated by certain substances released by cell damage and are also sensitised by certain chemical by-products of cell damage. Receptor subtypes exist for A-fibre and C-fibre nociceptors, and it is likely that there is some overlap in stimuli for activation between groups

Nomenclature can be complex and many sub-types of nociceptors have been described. Nociceptors are often classified into:

❖ *A-fibre nociceptors:* these help to detect stimuli with the potential to damage tissue and respond best to extremes of hot and cold, and to high intensity mechanical events. A-fibre nociceptor activity contributes to reflex responses (eg. withdrawal reflexes), and to 'first' or 'fast' pain sensations that help to locate the noxious stimuli (eg. 'pricking' and 'sharp' pain sensations, *Figure 2.10*). A-fibre nociceptors have been sub-classified into type 1 nociceptors, with a predominance of A-fibre mechano-heat nociceptors, and type 2 nociceptors, which are less responsive to mechanical stimuli. Both types of A-fibre nociceptor are likely to be sensitive to irritant chemicals.

❖ *C-fibre nociceptors:* these are particularly sensitive to chemicals released during actual cell damage such as hydrogen ions (H^+), potassium ions (K^+), serotonin (5-HT) and bradykinin. They also respond to noxious thermal and mechanical events. C-fibre nociceptor activity contributes to 'second' or 'slow' pain sensations that help to guard the injury from further damage (eg. 'dull' and 'aching' pain sensations, *Figure 2.10*). Significant proportions of C-fibre nociceptors are polymodal and can respond to thermal, mechanical, and chemical stimuli. It is now emerging that many A-fibre nociceptors are also polymodal (Raja *et al*, 1999; Drew and Wood, 2004; Koltzenburg, 2004).

It should be remembered that these subdivisions are gross oversimplifications. Furthermore, high intensity noxious stimuli will also activate non-nociceptive mechano and thermo receptors which have low thresholds of activation. Activity in these non-nociceptive mechano and thermo receptors will also 'flavour' the sensation of pain experienced by a person. In fact, when the nociceptive system becomes sensitised, these non-nociceptive receptors begin to signal noxious events.

Transmission

Afferent neurons transmit nerve impulses from nociceptors to the spinal cord and/or brainstem (peripheral transmission), and from the spinal cord and/or brainstem to higher centres in the brain (central transmission) (*Figure 2.10*) (Craig and Dostrovsky, 1999; Raja *et al*, 1999; Willis, 2004).

❖ *Peripheral transmission:* A-fibre nociceptors transmit impulses in small diameter myelinated A-delta afferents with conduction velocities above $2\,ms^{-1}$, usually in the $25\,ms^{-1}$ range. Impulses in these 'fast' transmitting nociceptive fibres reach the brain 'first' and contribute to the sharp, severe, localised pain immediately following a noxious event ('fast' or 'first' pain). C-fibre nociceptors transmit impulses in small diameter unmyelinated C afferents with conduction velocities below $2\,ms^{-1}$, usually in the $0.5\,ms^{-1}$ range. Impulses in these 'slow' transmitting nociceptive fibres reach the brain after the A-fibre impulses and contribute to the dull aching, less severe, spreading pain (ie. 'slow' or 'second' pain).

Most peripheral nociceptive afferents terminate in the superficial part of the dorsal horn and synapse directly or indirectly (via interneurons) on to central nociceptive transmission cells. Peripheral nociceptive afferents release a variety of excitatory substances, although all tend to use glutamate as their main neurotransmitter.

❖ *Central transmission:* central nociceptive transmission neurons transmit information about noxious stimuli from the spinal cord and brainstem to higher brain centres such as the thalamus (spinothalamic tracts [STT]), the brainstem reticular formation (spinoreticular tract [SRT]), and the hypothalamus and forebrain (spinohypothalamic tract [SHT]). Activity in central nociceptive transmission neurons is increased with input from nociceptive peripheral afferents and excitatory interneurons. When the nociceptive system is operating in its normal state, activity in central nociceptive transmission neurons is reduced (modulated), with input from low threshold (innocuous) mechano and thermal afferents (segmental modulation), and/ or descending pain inhibitory pathways arising from the brain (extrasegmental modulation). Interneuron-releasing inhibitory neurotransmitters, such as gamma-amino-butyric-acid (GABA), glycine and metenkephalin are often involved (see 'The suppressed pain state', *pp. 48–49*).

Central nociceptive transmission neurons can be categorised into nociceptive specific neurons (NS) and wide dynamic range neurons (WDR, *Figure 2.13*). NS neurons respond to high intensity stimuli and are predominantly found in lamina I of the dorsal horn. They send information in the spinothalamic tract which provides a rapid and direct route to sensory areas of the cerebrum (eg. somatosensory cortex). This provides information regarding the intensity, quality, and location of the noxious stimuli. WDR neurons respond to non-noxious and noxious stimuli arriving in A-fibre and C-fibre nociceptors and A-fibre 'touch' afferents. This is why they are called 'wide dynamic range' neurons. WDR neurons are predominantly found in lamina V of the dorsal horn and form multi-synaptic pathways projecting to the reticular formation in the brainstem and to the limbic system and the frontal lobes in the cerebrum. Central nociceptive transmission neurons also project to the hypothalamus via spinohypothalamic tracts to elicit sympathetic changes, as described earlier.

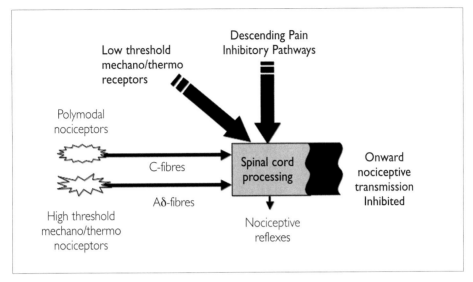

Figure 2.12: Endogenous pain suppression systems. Activity in low threshold mechanoreceptors (ie. touch and rubbing), and thermoreceptors (ie. cooling or warming), and descending pain inhibitory pathways will inhibit ongoing activity in central nociceptive transmission cells

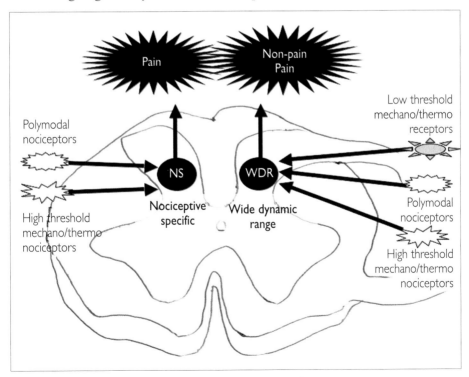

Figure 2.13: Central nociceptive transmission cells

Perception

Perception is the process by which we become aware of something through our senses. The primary somatosensory cortex of the cerebrum (SI) contributes to pain sensation by processing incoming information to aid discrimination of the location and nature of noxious and non-noxious stimuli impinging on the body. SI receives an ordered neural input of body parts from the opposite side of the body (*Figure 2.14*). Body parts with high densities of sensory receptor cells have proportionately larger areas of SI devoted to processing incoming information and are better at discriminating two discrete stimuli (ie. are more sensitive) (Penfield, 1968).

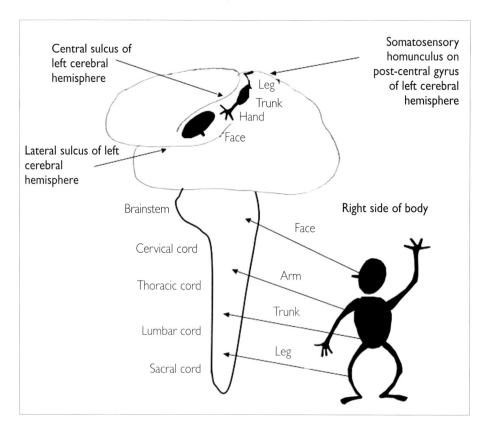

Figure 2.14: Somatotopic ('body map') representation in the central nervous system. Somatosensory pathways project in an ordered manner to areas of the contralateral somatosensory cortex (SI). Large areas of the cortex process input from body parts that have fine discrimination, creating a distorted body map termed a homunculus

Removal of nociceptive transmission neurons or removal of the somatosensory cortex itself does not improve pain in the long term, suggesting that pain perception is more complex than simply activating a single pain centre in the brain. Neuroimaging techniques, such as positron emission tomography (PET) and functional magnetic resonance imaging (fMRI) have revealed activity in a variety of brain areas when healthy humans experience experimentally-induced pain. Interestingly, different patterns of brain activity are seen in patients with persistent pain suggesting that there is no brain 'centre' devoted to pain experience, and that different areas become active in different situations. Areas commonly seen to be involved in pain processing are the thalamus and somatosensory cortex (sensory dimensions), the cingulate gyrus and insula (affective dimensions), and the prefrontal cortex (cognitive dimensions) (Gybels and Tasker, 1999; Ingvar and Hsieh, 1999; Davis, 2000; Treede *et al*, 2000).

Nociception — the sensitised pain state

Increased sensitivity to stimuli happens to cutaneous, visceral and muscle tissue and helps to protect the tissue from further damage. This sensitisation occurs in the periphery and in the central nervous system (*Figure 2.15*).

Peripheral sensitisation

Damage to cells causes the accumulation of algesic (pain producing) substances in the extracellular fluid which reduces the threshold of activation of nociceptors at the site of injury (peripheral sensitisation). These algesic substances have leaked out of damaged cells; have been synthesised from precursors that have themselves leaked out of damaged cells; or have arrived in the area as a result of plasma extravasation ('outside vessel') or lymphocyte migration.

In addition, nerve impulses generated by nociceptor activity invade the distal branches of the nociceptor free nerve endings, causing the release of substance P and other trophic chemicals into the surrounding tissue (*Figure 2.16*). Some of these chemicals may play a critical role in wound healing. This 'chemical soup' produces vasodilatation, increased blood flow, increased permeability of blood vessels, and plasma extravasation associated with inflamed tissue (ie. redness, heat, and swelling). Some algesic substances such as Bradykinin, 5-HT, H^+, and K^+ activate nociceptors leading to pain in the absence of external stimuli. Other substances, such as prostaglandins, leukotrienes, noradrenaline, adenosine, adenosine 5-triphosphate (ATP), and nitric oxide, sensitise nociceptors by lowering their threshold of activation (Levine and Reichling, 1999).

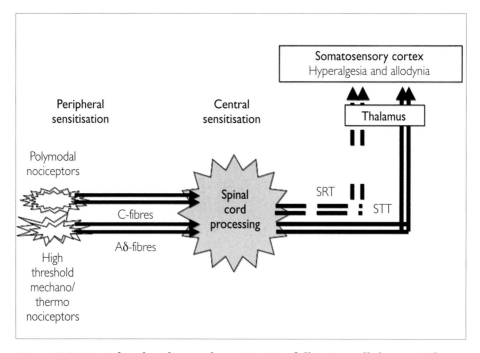

Figure 2.15: Peripheral and central sensitisation following cell damage. The thresholds of activation of peripheral and central nociceptive cells are lowered as a result of sensitisation causing an amplification of provoking stimuli

A basic knowledge of this neurobiology of peripheral sensitisation helps to understand how some pain-relieving drugs work. Non-steroidal anti-inflammatory drugs (NSAIDs, eg. ibuprofen, diclofenac, and aspirin) reduce the production of prostaglandins by inhibiting cyclo-oxygenase (Cox), an enzyme that speeds up the formation of prostaglandins (PG) from arachidonic acid. Cox exists as two isozymes (Cox-I and Cox-II), and drugs that selectively inhibit Cox-II were developed to reduce side-effects and improve efficacy. These

Cox-II inhibitors (eg. celecoxib, etodolac, rofecoxib and meloxicam) are used for short-term treatment of acute inflammation in joints caused by arthritis, but there has been concern about risks to the cardiovascular system. The effect of NSAIDs on bleeding and inflammation needs to be carefully evaluated prior to use for mild wound pain (Seibert *et al*, 1994).

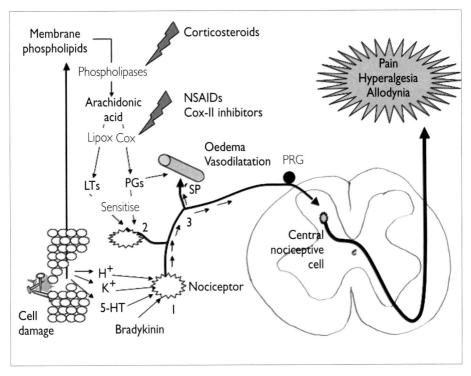

Figure 2.16: Peripheral events following tissue damage. Substances resulting from tissue damage can directly activate nociceptors [1] or can cause the synthesis of leukotrienes [LTs] and prostaglandins [PGs] that act to sensitise nociceptors [2]. Impulses also invade the nerve endings of the nociceptor and release substance P [SP]. This inflammatory soup causes vasodilatation and plasma extravasation [3]. Enzymes that catalyse the synthesis of LT and PG (ie. phospholipases, lipoxases [Lipox] and cyclo-oxygenases [Cox]) can be inhibited by corticosteroids, NSAIDs and Cox-II inhibitors. PRG = posterior root ganglion

Central sensitisation

Damage to cells resulting in persistent C-fibre nociceptor activity also reduces the threshold of activation of central nociceptive transmission cells (central sensitisation) through the process of 'wind-up'. Wind-up is a form of temporal summation whereby central nociceptive transmission neurons increase in their response to repeated C-fibre nociceptor activity, as would occur in post-burn or post-abrasion injuries. Wind-up contributes to hyperalgesia by making central nociceptive transmission neurons hyperexcitable and they may even begin to respond to non-noxious stimuli to produce allodynia (*Figure 2.17*). This is what makes wound dressing changes so unpleasant. Central nociceptive transmission neurons also expand their receptive fields so that they begin to respond to stimuli applied to sites on the body that do not normally activate the neuron producing secondary hyperalgesia. It is believed that secondary hyperalgesia in the healthy tissue that surrounds the injury is due to central sensitisation, rather than local accumulation of algesic substances at the site of damage (Cousins and Power, 1999; Doubell *et al*, 1999; Raja *et al*, 1999; Dickenson *et al*, 2004).

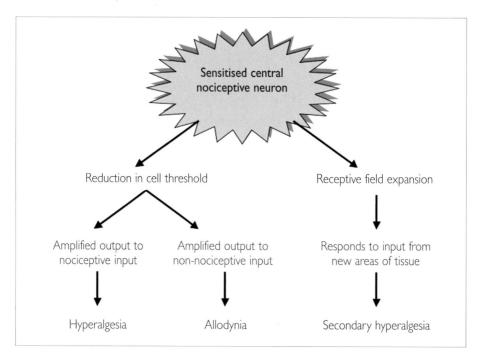

Figure 2.17: Characteristics of a sensitised central nociceptive cell

The pharmacology of central sensitisation is complex and involves many neurochemicals. Two common neurotransmitters released by peripheral nociceptive afferents on to central nociceptive transmission cells are glutamate, which is an excitatory amino acid and substance P, which is an excitatory peptide. These substances sensitise the central nociceptive transmission cell by binding to and activating a variety of membrane receptors such as NMDA (N-methyl D-aspartate) receptors (eg. glutamate), and neurokinin receptors (eg. substance P). Many other transmitter substances are also involved in central sensitisation such as calcitonin-gene-related-peptide (CGRP), somatostatin, vasoactive intestinal polypeptide (VIP), nerve growth factor, and nitric oxide (Yaksh, 1999).

The NMDA receptor may have a crucial role in the transition between acute and chronic pain (Dickenson and Sullivan, 1987). Activation of the NMDA receptor by sustained release of glutamate and substance P from peripheral nociceptive afferent terminals results in an influx of Ca^{++} into the central nociceptive transmission neuron (_Figure 2.18_). This changes the neuron's excitability and structure, and results in reorganisation of neuronal circuitry within the central nervous system (central neuroplasticity). Ketamine is a drug that acts as an NMDA antagonist and has been used to try to prevent central sensitisation occurring in pains due to severe burns. Furthermore, pre-emptive analgesics have also been used prior to surgical procedures to reduce potential long-term consequences of central sensitisation associated with post-operative pain.

Amplified pain resulting from treatments, such as wound dressing and debridement, are clear examples of allodynia and hyperalgesia and result from peripheral and central sensitisation. The importance of effectively managing pain during these procedures cannot be over emphasised, because failure to do so may result in persistent central sensitisation, which may be irreversible.

The persistent (chronic) pain state

A sensitised nociceptive system should return to its pre-sensitised state once tissue has healed and pain should disappear. However, many patients experience persistent pain. This may occur before the formation of a wound, in non-healing wounds, or after a wound has healed. Persistent pain may be nociceptive (ie. via activation of nociceptors), neuropathic (ie. when there has been nerve damage), or both.

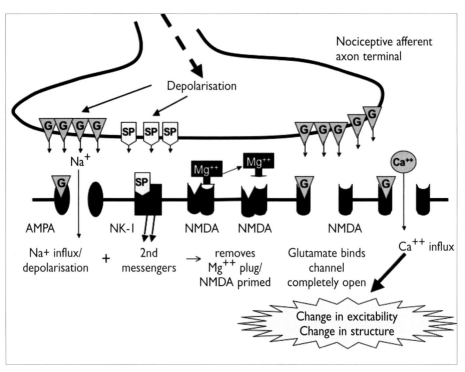

Figure 2.18: Activation of NMDA receptors. Depolarisation of the nociceptor afferent terminal causes the release of glutamate [G] and substance P [SP], either from separate fibres or co-released by the same fibre. Glutamate activates AMPA receptors and depolarises the central nociceptive neuron, whereas substance P activates neurokinin receptors [NK-1] activating second messengers. Simultaneous activation of AMPA and NK-1 receptors removes an Mg^{++} plug from the NMDA receptor and, if glutamate activates the NMDA receptor, Ca^{++} channels will open. An influx of Ca^{++} to the post synaptic central nociceptive cell leads to long-term changes in the structural and functional abilities of the central nociceptive cell

Persistent nociceptive pain

Nociceptive wound pain is more common than neuropathic wound pain and, as described previously, results from ongoing activation and sensitisation of nociceptors. Persistent nociceptive pain may be due to an underlying condition causing ongoing ischaemia, oedema, or tissue damage, as seen with arterial and venous disease. Alternatively, it may result from the prolonged time for healing of a serious trauma such as a post-burn injury, whereby peripheral and central sensitisation will persist and the wound will be sensitive to provoking stimuli. Nociceptive wound pain is receptive to primary analgesic agents such as paracetamol, NSAIDs, local anaesthetics, and opioids. Failure to manage the pain may cause long-term changes in the structural and functional organisation of the nociceptive system, so that pain persists even if the wound eventually heals.

In situations where there has been nerve damage, pain may persist despite the apparent healing of tissue, as seen with post-amputation pain or post-herpetic neuralgia. In these circumstances, pain may result from pathophysiology of the nociceptive system.

Neuropathic pain

Pain resulting from nerve damage is called neuropathic pain. Nerve lesions may affect sensory, motor and autonomic fibre symptoms and, as a consequence, response to treatment can be variable. Factors contributing to neuropathic pain include:

- hypersensitive central nociceptive cells
- abnormal inputs to central nociceptive cells
- reflex muscle spasm
- ectopic impulse generation
- loss of large diameter afferent (segmental) inhibition.

There may also be sympathetic hyperactivity (Devor and Seltzer, 1999; Hansson *et al*, 2001). However, persistent central sensitisation seems to be a common factor following injury to neural tissue.

In general, neuropathic pain is characterised by unusual sensations such as numbness, paraesthesia, and pains that are described as shooting, burning, electrical, and deep aching. Mechanical and/or thermal allodynia and hyperalgesia may be present. Neuropathic wound pain is difficult to control and antidepressant or anti-epileptic drugs are commonly used.

Lesions of peripheral nerves, as seen in diabetes or in deep wounds, are termed peripheral neuropathies. If nerves are severed distal to the cell body, a clump of regenerating neuronal sprouts termed a neuroma may form. The neuroma, and the posterior root ganglion, may be spontaneously active (ie. ectopic firing) producing pain in the absence of stimuli (*Figure 2.19*). Neuromas are also sensitive to provoking stimuli and may generate excessive amounts of nerve impulses which further sensitise central nociceptive transmission neurons. This may explain why some wounds that appear to have healed, may still be painful to touch, as seen in post-amputation stump pain (Wall and Gutnick, 1974; Dickenson *et al*, 2001).

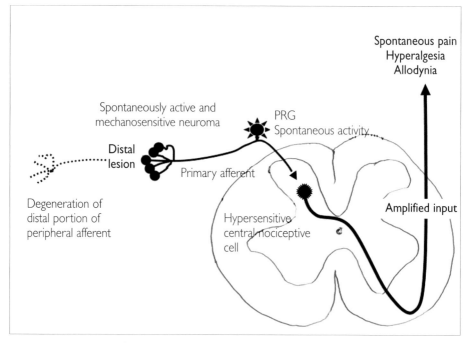

Figure 2.19: Nerve lesions distal to the posterior root ganglion. Distal lesions cause ectopic impulse generation at neuroma and the posterior root ganglion [PRG] leading to central sensitisation

When nerves are damaged proximal to the cell body, central nociceptive transmission neurons may become spontaneously active because of the lack of normal afferent input (*Figure 2.20*). This may explain why an injury that appears to have healed may still generate background pain, as seen following brachial plexus avulsions when a person's arm is paralysed and insensitive to touch, yet manifests a severe aching pain. Phantom limb pains are also likely to result in part from spontaneously active central nociceptive transmission neurons (Devor and Seltzer, 1999).

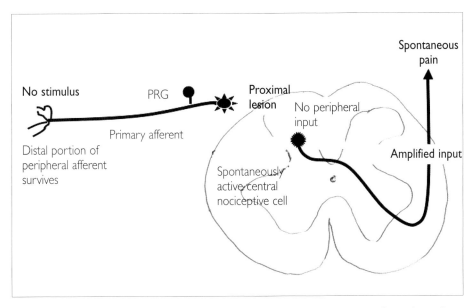

Figure 2.20: Nerve lesions proximal to the posterior root ganglion (PRG). Ectopic impulse generation arises in central nociceptive cells due to the lack of peripheral input

Reorganisation of central neuronal circuits

One consequence of nerve damage is structural and functional reorganisation of the nervous system. For example, areas of SI with input from intact nerves invade areas of SI that have lost their input due to nerve damage. This may explain some of the unusual phantom sensations experienced post amputation, such as stroking the cheek with a Q-tip generating a phantom hand sensation. This is because the area of SI receiving input from the cheek invades the neighbouring area of SI which has lost its normal input from the amputated hand (Flor *et al*, 1995; Flor *et al*, 1998; Montoya *et al*, 1998).

Neuropathy with diminished sensation

Sometimes tissue does not heal, yet there is no pain because nerve damage has caused diminished sensation, as seen with neuropathic foot ulcers (neuropathy with diminished sensation). Peripheral neuropathy, as seen with diabetes, can result in sensory loss causing ulceration at sites of high pressure. Neuropathies of motor and autonomic nerves may cause abnormal plantar pressure and anhydrotic skin which is prone to fissuring, resulting in neuropathic foot ulcers. Interestingly, neuropathic foot ulcers are often painless despite the potential for peripheral and central sensitisation (Edmonds and Foster, 2006).

The suppressed pain state — pain modulation

Pain sensation can be reduced by suppressing activity in the nociceptive system, as described by the Gate Control Theory of Pain (Melzack and Wall, 1965). The 'pain gate' is a metaphor to explain regulation of nociceptive information. The 'pain gate' can be opened by activity in peripheral nociceptor transmission pathways (A-fibre and C-fibre nociceptors), leading to onward transmission of noxious information to the brain. When the 'pain gate' is closed, onward transmission of noxious information from the spinal cord to the brain is suppressed. This can be achieved in two ways (*Figure 2.21*).

Activity in non-noxious afferents (segmental modulation)

Activity in peripheral non-noxious afferents (eg. touch and pressure) can be generated by rubbing healthy skin close to painful or damaged areas of the body, hence the term 'rubbing pain better'. Passing low intensity electrical currents across the skin can also be used to activate non-noxious afferents in a technique called transcutaneous electrical nerve stimulation (TENS). In many respects, TENS 'electrically rubs pain better'. It has been shown that TENS reduces central nociceptive transmission neurons by activating inhibitory interneurons in the spinal cord that release GABA and enkephalins (Garrison and Foreman, 1994; Johnson, 2002; Sluka and Walsh, 2003).

Activity in descending pain inhibitory nerve pathways (extrasegmental modulation)

Activity in neural pathways arising from areas in the brainstem, such as the periaqueductal grey (PAG) and the raphe nuclei, causes inhibition of central nociceptive transmission neurons through pre- and post-synaptic inhibitory mechanisms (*Figure 2.21*). These descending pain inhibitory nerve pathways involve many transmitter substances including opioid peptides (predominantly acting on µ receptors, but also on δ and κ receptors), serotonin, and noradrenaline (acting on α–2 receptors). These receptors are prime targets for many analgesic drugs such as opioids (eg. morphine) and amitryptiline (Fields and Basbaum, 1999; Dubner and Ren, 2004; Villanueva and Fields, 2004).

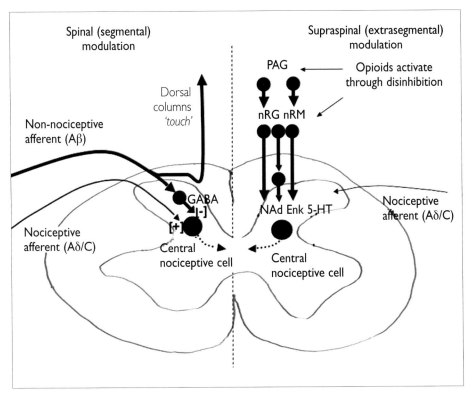

Figure 2.21: Endogenous pain suppression systems. Ongoing activity in central nociceptive transmission cells can be reduced by inhibitory interneurons [-] releasing GABA and possibly met-enkephalin [Enk] at a segmental level, or by activity in the periaqueductal gray [PAG], nucleus raphe magnus [nRM] and nucleus raphe gigantocellularis [nRG] at an extrasegmental level releasing noradrenalin [NAd], 5-hydroxytryptamine [5-HT] and enkephalin [Enk]. Excitatory = [+]; Inhibitory = [-]

Deep structures and referred pain

Nociceptors in deep structures

Most knowledge about pain physiology comes from studies on superficial structures like the skin. However, wounds may penetrate deeper somatic structures, such as skeletal muscle, connective tissue of the joints and bone. Wounds may also penetrate visceral structures, such as cardiac muscle and smooth muscle of the gastrointestinal, renal and vascular systems. Nociceptors in the skin evolved to signal encounters with external stimuli and tend to generate discrete localised pains, promoting escape behaviour. Nociceptors in deep tissue have evolved to detect noxious stimuli resulting from stretching and imbalances in fluid pH, and they tend to generate pain that is dull and less well localised, as characterised in *Table 2.3*.

Table 2.3: The characteristics of pain arising from superficial versus deep tissue (adapted from Cousins, 1987)		
	Superficial	**Deep**
Tissues	Cutaneous, mucous	Cardiac, skeletal and smooth muscle. Fascia, periosteum, joint and connective tissue
Intensity of pain	Often related to severity of damage	Diminished relationship to severity of damage
Quality of pain	Sharp, pricking, stinging	Dull, sore, aching
Location of pain	Precise and localised Strong relationship with stimulus/injury	Diffuse and poorly localised Weaker relationship with stimulus/injury and may be referred to another area of the body
Temporal aspects of pain	Often constant rather than periodic	Often periodic and may build to peak intensity
Related symptoms	Autonomic symptoms occur if damage is moderate and involves deep tissue	Autonomic symptoms often present — nausea, vomiting, sweating, palpitations

The principles of nociception are similar for deep structures as they are for the skin. A-fibre and C-fibre nociceptors become sensitised in the presence of tissue damage and contribute to spontaneous pain, allodynia and hyperalgesia. However, nociceptors in deeper structures vary considerably in the type of stimuli that provoke activity. Skeletal muscle is sensitive to contraction in the presence of ischaemia, which can generate a deep aching pain, as seen with limb ischaemia and associated ischaemic ulcers. These pains can have both nociceptive and neuropathic elements. Visceral structures are sensitive to twisting, distension and chemical irritants (eg. stomach acid), but are relatively insensitive to cutting, heat or pinching (Cousins, 1987; Blendis, 1999; Procacci *et al*, 1999; Mense and Simons, 2001).

Physiology of referred pain

The poor localisation of deep somatic and visceral pain is due to fewer central nociceptive transmission neurons dedicated to visceral input. Damage in deep structures may result in referred pain which is felt at sites remote from tissue damage and pathology. Pathology in deep structures often produces characteristic patterns of skin sensitivity and pain because their afferents are bundled in nerves that primarily innervate structures like the skin. Often pain is referred to the cutaneous area innervated by the same spinal segment (dermatome) as the visceral structure, because visceral and cutaneous afferents supply the same central nociceptive transmission neuron (*Figure 2.22*). The brain interprets the afferent input as arising from cutaneous structures because of the higher proportion of cutaneous afferents converging on central nociceptive transmission neurons. Referred pain can confuse the clinician and the patient (Fields, 1987).

Summary

Wound pain is a major factor issue for patients and may be associated with underlying pathology and/or treatment, such as debridement or dressing changes. Under-treatment of wound pain is a problem and leads to a state of physiological stress which is detrimental to health. Nowadays, the concept of pain being generated by a 'hard wired pain pathway' is outdated, as many biopsychosocial factors influence the way that we experience pain. The neural circuitry that detects stimuli that produce actual or potential tissue damage is called the nociceptive system. In its normal state, the nociceptive system detects noxious stimuli and generates protective reflex responses and pain so that we can avoid the noxious stimuli in the future. In its suppressed state, the nociceptive system reduces pain to enable us to escape from threatening situations even if there is appreciable tissue damage. In its sensitised state, the nociceptive system amplifies pain and this aids tissue healing by discouraging behaviours that may cause further tissue damage. Some pain-relieving treatments try to block nociceptive information reaching the brain by interfering with the nociceptive system. NSAIDs and local anaesthetics are good examples. Some pain-relieving treatments interact with our own endogenous pain-relieving systems. Opioids and TENS are good examples. Persistent wound pain may be nociceptive in origin, resulting from ongoing activation of nociceptors and sensitisation of the nociceptive system. This may be due to an underlying condition or a prolonged time for a wound to heal. Persistent wound pain may be neuropathic in origin, resulting from damage to nerves. It will cause irreversible functional and structural reorganisation in the nervous system.

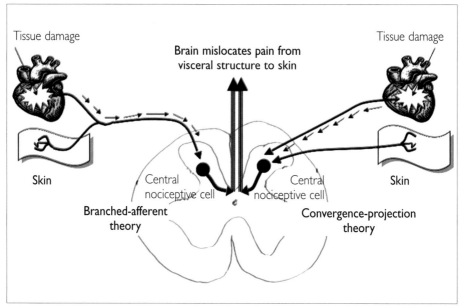

Figure 2.22: The physiology of referred pain. The brain is unable to discriminate the source of the incoming noxious information [arrows] as arising from visceral structures (eg. heart) or somatic structures (eg. skin). This tends to result in pain referred to the somatic structures

References

Baron R, Janig W (2004) The role of the sympathetic nervous system in pain processing. In: Villanueva L, Dickenson AH, Ollat H, eds. *The Pain System in Normal and Pathological States: A Primer for Clinicians' Progress. Pain Research and Management, Volume 31.* IASP Press, Seattle: 193–210

Basbaum A (2004) Molecular approaches to understanding the anatomical substrates of nociceptive processing. In: Villanueva L, Dickenson AH, Ollat H, eds. *The Pain System in Normal and Pathological States: A Primer for Clinicians' Progress. Pain Research and Management, Volume 31.* IASP Press, Seattle: 123–137.

Blendis LM (1999) Abdominal pain. In: Wall PD, Melzack R, eds. *Textbook of Pain.* Churchill Livingstone, Edinburgh: 603–19

Cousins M (1987) Visceral disease. In: Andersson S, Bond M, Mehta M, Swerdlow M, eds. *Chronic Non-cancer Pain.* MTP Press Limited, Lancaster: 119–30

Cousins M, Power I (1999) Acute and post-operative pain. In: Wall PD, Melzack R, eds. *Textbook of Pain.* Churchill Livingstone, Edinburgh: 447–92

Craig AD, Dostrovsky JO (1999) Medulla to thalamus. In: Wall PD, Melzack R, eds. *Textbook of Pain.* Churchill Livingstone, Edinburgh: 183–214

Davis KD (2000) Studies of pain using functional magnetic resonance imaging. In: Casey KL, Bushnell MC, eds. *Pain Imaging. Pain Research and Management, Volume 18.* IASP Press, Seattle: 195–210

Devor M, Seltzer Z (1999) Pathophysiology of damaged nerves in relation to chronic pain. In: Wall PD, Melzack R, eds. *Textbook of Pain.* Churchill Livingstone, Edinburgh: 129–64

Dickenson AH, Sullivan AF (1987) Evidence for a role of the NMDA receptor in the frequency dependent potentiation of deep rat dorsal horn nociceptive neurones following C fibre stimulation. *Neuropharmacol* 26: 1235–8

Dickenson AH, Matthews EA, Suzuki R (2001) Central nervous system mechanisms of pain in peripheral neuropathy. In: Hansson PT, Fields HL, Hill RG, Marchettini P, eds. *Neuropathic Pain: Pathophysiology and Treatment. Pain Research and Management, Volume 21.* IASP Press, Seattle: 85–106

Dickenson AH, Suzuki R, Matthews EA, Rahman W, Urch C, Seagrove L, Rygh L (2004) Balancing excitations and inhibitions in the spinal circuits. In: Villanueva L, Dickenson AH, Ollat H, eds. *The Pain System in Normal and Pathological States: A Primer for Clinicians' Progress. Pain Research and Management Volume 31*. IASP Press, Seattle: 79–105

Doubell TP, Mannion RJ, Woolf CJ (1999) The dorsal horn: state-dependent sensory process, plasticity and the generation of pain. In: Wall PD, Melzack R, eds. *Textbook of Pain*. Churchill Livingstone, Edinburgh: 165–82

Drew LJ, Wood JN (2004) Molecular mechanisms of noxious mechanosensation. In: Villanueva L, Dickenson AH, Ollat H, eds. *The Pain System in Normal and Pathological States: A Primer for Clinicians' Progress. Pain Research and Management, Volume 31*. IASP Press, Seattle: 3–27

Dubner R, Ren K (2004) Brainstem modulation of pain after inflammation. In: Villanueva L, Dickenson AH, Ollat H, eds. *The Pain System in Normal and Pathological States: A Primer for Clinicians' Progress. Pain Research and Management, Volume 31*. IASP Press, Seattle: 107–22

Edmonds ME, Foster AVM (2006) Diabetic foot ulcers. *Br Med J* **332**: 407–10

Fields HL (1987) Pain from deep tissues and referred pain. In: Fields HL, ed. *Pain*. McGraw-Hill Book Company, New York: 79–97

Fields HL, Basbaum AI (1999) Central nervous system mechanisms of pain modulation. In: Wall PD, Melzack R, eds. *Textbook of Pain*. Churchill Livingstone, Edinburgh: 309–30

European Wound Management Association (EWMA) (2002) *Position Document: Pain at wound dressing changes*. Medical Education Partnership Ltd, London

Flor, H, Elbert T, Knecht S (1995) Phantom-limb pain as a perceptual correlate of cortical reorganization following arm amputation. *Nature* **375**: 482–4

Flor H, Elbert T, Muhlnickel W (1998) Cortical reorganization and phantom phenomena in congenital and traumatic upper-extremity amputees. *Exp Brain Res* **119**: 205–12

Garrison DW, Foreman RD (1994) Decreased activity of spontaneous and noxiously evoked dorsal horn cells during transcutaneous electrical nerve stimulation (TENS). *Pain* **58**: 309–15

Gybels JM, Tasker RR (1999) Central neurosurgery. In: Wall PD, Melzack R, eds. *Textbook of Pain*. Churchill Livingstone, Edinburgh: 1307–39

Hansson PT, Lacerenza M, Marchettini (2001) Aspects of clinical and experimental pain: The clinical perspective. In: Hansson PT, Fields HL, Hill RG, Marchettini P, eds. *Neuropathic Pain: Pathophysiology and treatment. Pain Research and Management, Volume 21*. IASP Press, Seattle: 1–18

Ingvar M, Hsieh JC (1999) The image of pain. In: Wall PD, Melzack R, eds. *Textbook of Pain*. Churchill Livingstone, Edinburgh: 215–33

Johnson MI (2002) Transcutaneous electrical nerve stimulation. In: Kitchen SM, ed. *Electrotherapy: Evidence-based practice*. Churchill Livingstone, Edinburgh: 259–86

Levine JD, Reichling DB (1999) Peripheral mechanisms of inflammatory pain. In: Wall PD, Melzack R, eds. *Textbook of Pain*. Churchill Livingstone, Edinburgh: 59–84

Koltzenburg M (2004) Thermal sensitivity of sensory neurons. In: Villanueva L, Dickenson AH, Ollat H, eds. *The Pain System in Normal and Pathological States: A Primer for Clinicians' Progress. Pain Research and Management, Volume 31*. IASP Press, Seattle: 29–43

Krasner D (1995) The chronic wound experience. *Ostomy/Wound Management* **41**: 20–5

McCaffery M (1983) *Nursing the Patient in Pain*. Harper & Row, London

Melzack R (1975) The McGill Pain Questionnaire: major properties and scoring methods. *Pain* **1**: 277–99

Melzack R, Katz J (1999) Pain measurements in persons in pain. In: Wall PD, Melzack R, eds. *Textbook of Pain*. Churchill Livingstone, Edinburgh: 409–26

Melzack R, Wall P (1965) Pain mechanisms: A new theory. *Science* **150**: 971–9

Melzack R, Wall PD (1988) *The Challenge of Pain*. Penguin Books, London

Mense S, Simons D (2001) *Muscle Pain. Understanding its nature, diagnosis, and treatment*. Lippincott Williams and Wilkins, Philadelphia

Merskey H, Bogduk N (1994) *Classification of Chronic Pain: Descriptions of Chronic Pain Syndromes and Definitions of Pain Terms*. 2nd edn. IASP Press, Seattle

Moffat CJ, Franks PJ, Hollingworth H (2002) Understanding wound pain and trauma: an international perspective. In: *European Wound Management Association Position Document. Pain at wound dressing changes*. Medical Education Partnership Limited, London: 2–7

Montoya P, Ritter K, Huse E, Larbig W, Braun C, Topfner S *et al* (1998) The cortical somatotopic map and phantom phenomena in subjects with congenital limb atrophy and traumatic amputees with phantom limb pain. *Eur J Neurosci* **10**: 1095–102

Penfield W (1968) Engrams in the human brain. Mechanisms of memory. *Proc R Soc Med* **61**: 831–40

Procacci P, Zoppi M, Maresca M (1999) Heart, vascular and haemopathic pain. In: Wall PD, Melzack R, eds. *Textbook of Pain*. Churchill Livingstone, Edinburgh: 621–40

Raja SN, Meyer RA, Ringkamp M *et al* (1999) Peripheral neural mechanisms of nociception. In: Wall PD, Melzack R, eds. *Textbook of Pain*. Churchill Livingstone, Edinburgh: 11–58

Ready L, Edwards WT (1992) *Management of Acute Pain: A practical guide*. IASP Press, Seattle.

Seibert K, Zhang Y, Leahy K *et al* (1994) Pharmacological and biochemical demonstration of the role of cyclooxygenase 2 in inflammation and pain. *Proc Natl Acad Sci USA* **91**: 12013–7

Sluka KA, Walsh D (2003) Transcutaneous electrical nerve stimulation: basic science mechanisms and clinical effectiveness. *J Pain* 4(3): 109–21

Treede RD, Apkarian AV, Bromm B (2000) Cortical representation of pain: functional characterization of nociceptive areas near the lateral sulcus. *Pain* 87: 113–19

Villanueva L, Fields HL (2004) Endogenous central mechanisms of pain modulation. In: Villanueva L, Dickenson AH, Ollat H, eds. *The Pain System in Normal and Pathological States: A Primer for Clinicians' Progress. Pain Research and Management, Volume 31*. IASP Press, Seattle: 223–46

Willis WD (2004) Spinothalamocortical Processing of Pain. In: Villanueva L, Dickenson AH, Ollat H, eds. *The Pain System in Normal and Pathological States: A Primer for Clinicians Progress. Pain Research and Management, Volume 31*. IASP Press, Seattle: 155–78

Wall PD, Gutnick M (1974) Properties of afferent nerve impulses originating from a neuroma. *Nature* **248**: 740–3

Woolf CJ (1987) Physiological, inflammatory and neuropathic pain. *Adv Tech Stand Neurosurg* **15**: 39-62.

Woolf CJ (1994) The dorsal horn: state-dependent sensory processing and the generation of pain. In: Wall PD, Melzack R, eds. *Textbook of Pain*. Churchill Livingstone, Edinburgh: 101–12

Woolf CJ, Salter MW (2000) Neuronal plasticity: increasing the gain in pain. *Science* **288**: 1765–9

Yaksh T (1999) Central pharmacology of nociceptive transmission. In: Wall PD, Melzack R, eds. *Textbook of Pain*. Churchill Livingstone, Edinburgh: 253–308

Section II: Pain at dressing change

CHAPTER 3

SKIN TRAUMA

Pauline Beldon

The current UK population is 59.8 million, 16% of which are aged 65 years and older, within which the proportion of those aged 85 years and older is now 12% (Department of Health [DoH], 2004). The elderly population often have comorbidities resulting in an increase in skin and soft tissue traumatic injuries.

The skin is unquestionably a vital organ and, since its structure and function are inextricably linked, it is inevitable that structural changes due to ageing will lead to functional impairment (Grove, 1986). The skin continues to perform the functions of; absorption, excretion, protection, secretion, thermoregulation, pigment production, sensory perception and immunity (Butcher and White, 2005) but, due to ageing, does so less efficiently (Richey *et al*, 1988). Unfortunately, many age-related changes in the skin increase the propensity for skin trauma (*Table 3.1*). To protect the skin and manage skin trauma, it is important to understand these changes.

Age-related skin changes

Ageing leads to generalised atrophy of the skin causing it to become increasingly fragile and prone to trauma. Understanding these structural changes and their relation to the impaired function of the skin, helps in the management of a range of complex epidermal/dermal injuries.

Table 3.1: Age-related changes in skin
• Epidermis is thinner and flatter, uneven distribution of melanocytes leading to uneven pigmentation
• Flattening of the dermal-epidermal junction; increasing susceptibility to friction/shear forces, resulting in blistering and minor injuries
• Dermis has decreased bulk due to collagen atrophy
• Skin becomes wrinkled due to depletion of elastic fibres
• Decreased capillary loops in the dermis increase dangers of both hypo- and hyperthermia
• Decreased cutaneous sensitivity leads to increased danger of injury

Epidermis

With ageing, the epidermis becomes thinner and flatter, the basal keratinocytes become more cuboidal, rather than columnar, and the rate of keratinocyte proliferation is decreased (Smith, 1989). There is also a decrease in the numbers of melanocytes and, although these are still stimulated by sunlight to produce pigment, such response is diminished. The uneven distribution of heavily-pigmented cells increases with age, contributing to pigmented spots commonly seen on elderly skin, eg. liver spots (Fenske and Conard, 1988), and the elderly are at increased risk of sun-induced skin carcinoma (Smith, 1989).

Langerhans cells, which are antigen-producing cells within the immune system in the skin, decrease in numbers (Gilchrist *et al*, 1982), resulting in an impaired immune response and an increase in autoimmune disorders. There is an increased risk of skin disorders, such as epidermolysis bullosa (EB), bullous pemphoid and pemphigus, all of which disrupt the epidermis or dermal-epidermal junction (Smith, 1989), leading to blistering and multiple areas of skin trauma.

Dermal-epidermal junction

Perhaps one of the most important changes is the flattening of the dermal-epidermal junction. In young individuals there is a close interdigitation between the epidermis (rete pegs or ridges) and the dermis (dermal papillae) (Montagna and Carlisle, 1979). In the elderly, the dermal-epidermal junction is flattened due to loss of rete pegs and corresponding dermal papillae, which results in progressive loss of epidermal–dermal contact (Lavker, 1979), predisposing the individual to friction/shear injuries which often cause the separation of the epidermis from the underlying dermis, and resultant minor skin trauma (Fenske and Conard, 1988).

Dermis

The dermis is organised into the papillary, intermediate, and deep reticular dermis. The papillary dermis is the zone of greatest interaction between the epidermis and the dermis. It is more cellular, has finer, fibrous components and has a rich vascular supply (Smith, 1989). With age, the deep reticular dermis shows decreased cellularity and vascularity, and increased density of collagen and elastic fibres; the total amount of collagen is decreased and, as a result, the amount of reticular dermis is dramatically decreased. Consequently, the skin may be thinned by as much as 20% (Shuster *et al*, 1975).

In addition, the fine elastic fibres in the papillary dermis are depleted or entirely lost, and those within the reticular dermis mat together and become frayed. Together, the loss of collagen and dramatic loss or changes in elastic fibres result in elderly skin which is sagging and wrinkled, with poor elastic recoil following stretching, as seen when the elderly skin is stretched and torn when trying to struggle into tight-fitting clothes.

There are decreased numbers of capillary loops in the papillary dermis, corresponding to a flattening of the dermal papillae. This results in reduced microcirculation and, consequently, an impaired supply of nutrients and oxygen to the epidermis (Braverman and Fonferko, 1982). A decrease in vascularity, together with generalised loss of subcutaneous tissue, makes the elderly more prone to hypothermia. Conversely, the elderly are also susceptible to hyperthermia as blood cannot be sufficiently diverted to the skin when the ambient temperature rises. The decreased number of eccrine sweat glands in the dermis also contribute to the risk of hyperthermia (Foster *et al*, 1976).

Pacini's and Meissner's corpuscles, the cutaneous end organs responsible for pressure and light touch sensation respectively, gradually decrease with age to approximately a third of their original density. This decrease in cutaneous sensitivity might explain the increased prevalence of burn and other injuries in the elderly (Procacci *et al*, 1970; Solomon and Virtue, 1975).

Skin tears/avulsion injuries

Skin tears or simple avulsion injuries are traumatic wounds commonly seen in the elderly, often resulting from friction/shear. The most common sites for injury include; the dorsal aspect of the hands, forearms, elbows, knees, and the pre-tibial region of the lower legs. In the young, these areas have little subcutaneous or deep tissue protection, which decreases further with ageing. Hasty removal of adhesive wound dressings, or dressings with an adhesive border, may also cause skin trauma in the elderly (Thomas, 2003).

It is difficult to determine the prevalence of such injuries, as many are small and self-managed. Only the larger, more painful or infected injuries are brought to the attention of a healthcare professional via the GP surgery or A&E department. One retrospective review of incident reports over one year in a 703 residential care setting, highlighted that of a total of 1397 fall-related injuries, 533 were bruises and skin tears. In addition, of 1631 injuries reported not related to falls, 1562 were bruises and skin tears (Gurwitz *et al*, 1994). This high incidence further highlights the danger for the elderly with frail skin.

Risk assessment of skin tears

Guidelines for the management of skin tears in the elderly have been suggested by Baranoski (2001), Camp-Sorrel (1991), Cuzzell (1990, 2002) and Murray (2005). All have highlighted the need for thorough risk assessment of the individual as a means of trauma prevention. White *et al* (1994) noted three groups of elderly individuals who were most likely to sustain skin trauma, namely:

1. Those who were totally dependent upon others for all activities of daily living, including manual handling and repositioning in bed.

Individuals who were aggressively resistant to hands-on care most frequently sustained skin tears.

2. Independently mobile individuals with oedema to lower extremities who were injured while being transferred in/out of wheelchairs, the bath and while dressing.
3. Those with sight impairment, who sustained injuries going through doorways, or hitting against stationary equipment and furnishings.

White *et al* (1994) suggested a skin integrity risk assessment related to trauma. This highlighted to staff in a nursing home the vulnerability of the client group, which initially, as awareness was raised, increased the number of skin tears reported.

Table 3.2: Factors increasing the risk of skin trauma
• Medication — the long-term corticosteroid therapy
• Senile dementia/cognitive impairment
• Loss of mobility; being reliant on others for repositioning
• Involuntary movements
• Elderly, fragile skin
• Extreme debilitation
• Visual impairment (Nazarko, 2005)
• Co-morbidity — respiratory/cardiac failure, oedematous lower limbs

Skin trauma prevention strategies for the elderly

For the elderly to guard against skin trauma, they need to be made aware of the danger, and part of every healthcare professional's role is that of health promotion (Nursing and Midwifery Council [NMC], 2004). Verbal and written information may be necessary to ensure comprehension, and the necessity to involve family and carers should not be underestimated.

Maintaining a healthy, hydrated skin is not easy for the elderly. In addition to the changes in skin anatomy, the elderly are less disposed towards the same healthy appetite and fluid intake that they may have exhibited 30 years earlier. Indeed, many of the elderly admitted to hospital are nutritionally depleted (Pichard *et al*, 2004). Reduced skin hydration may predispose towards skin trauma. Consequently, it is important that the elderly are well hydrated, which can be difficult with a reduction in the thirst reflex (Stout *et al*, 1999).

A lifetime habit of washing with soap and water can be difficult to change, but elderly patients need to be aware that soaps are astringent in nature, and so are likely to cause further drying of the skin, increasing the risk of skin trauma (Penzer and Finch, 2001). Using an emollient instead of soap can protect the skin and help to prevent insensible loss of moisture.

Wearing fleece-lined jogging bottoms and knee-length socks can help protect the pre-tibial area from injury. Likewise, wearing clothes a size larger makes dressing easier, and helps to prevent tears to the skin on the arms/hands. Well-fitting, supportive shoes with slip-free soles also reduces the risk of falling (White *et al*, 1994).

Prevention of skin trauma in a care setting

If a patient has been identified as being at risk from skin trauma, it is important to take steps to minimise the risk. The following factors should be considered:

* Using appropriate equipment for repositioning patients to reduce friction/shear forces, ie. slide sheets. Never use the sheet under the patient, this will drag the skin and contribute to trauma.
* Ensuring that all staff understand why the elderly are at risk from skin trauma, and the importance of careful handling of the patient. In extreme cases, just grasping the patient too firmly will result in trauma.
* Avoiding the use of adhesive tape to the skin following blood tests as, on removal, they may cause skin trauma.
* Increased vigilance of the disorientated patient.
* Using padded wheelchair leg and foot plates and arm supports, cotside bumpers (when appropriate) may reduce the risk of injury.

* Suggesting to at-risk patients that they wear long-sleeved shirts and trousers to protect their limbs. Padded trousers are now commercially available to avoid lower limb trauma.
* Substituting soap with an emollient for washing. Also, patting the body dry rather than rubbing.
* Consider how often a patient is washed, do very elderly patients usually have a full body wash every day at home? Question whether the care setting's routine is being imposed on the patient.
* Keeping the environment well-lit and uncluttered reduces the risk of injury.
* Ensuring that doors to toilets are easy to open, thus reducing both the effort needed and the risk of overbalancing.

(Adapted from Baranoski, 2000)

Treatment of skin tears in the elderly

This is related to the classification of the skin tear (*Table 3.3*), the site and extent of the injury, together with the need to provide a comfortable wound dressing for the individual. Few studies have been reported addressing the difficulties in managing skin trauma wounds in the elderly (Edwards *et al*, 1998; Thomas *et al*, 1999; Meuleneire, 2002). Edwards *et al* (1998) reported a pilot study which compared four dressings; a transparent film (Opsite®, Smith & Nephew), a thin hydrocolloid (DuoDERM® Extra Thin, ConvaTec), a foam (Lyofoam®, Mölnlycke Health Care), and a combination of Steri-Strip™ Adhesive Skin Closures (3M™) and a non-adhesive cellulose polyester material dressing (Melolite®, Smith & Nephew). This study appeared to demonstrate that those individuals treated with non-occlusive dressings healed more quickly than those treated with occlusive dressings. However, the study does not state the severity of skin tears that had been sustained, or their size, or whether all skin tears included in the study were considered to be the same classification of injury, calling into question the results. Thomas *et al* (1999) studied 37 subjects with category II or category III skin tears. The subjects were allocated either an opaque foam dressing or a transparent film dressing. The results revealed that 94% of the subjects treated with the foam dressing experienced complete healing, compared with 65% of the subjects who were treated with the film dressing. It is questionable whether category II tears, which involve loss of the epidermis alone, can be compared with category III tears, which include loss of dermal tissue, since the latter will take far longer to heal. Meuleneire (2002) did not perform a comparative study, but examined the use of a silicone-coated net dressing (Mepitel®, Mölnlycke Health Care) in category I and II skin tears. Meuleneire (2002) discovered that 83% of the patients' wounds had healed within eight days. Although a comparative dressing was not examined, this study is important because Meuleneire (2002) drew attention to the practicality of treatment of skin tear wounds, highlighting that use of adhesive dressings, such as hydrocolloids, films, or adhesive strips, can further traumatise the skin on removal. Moreover, the use of adhesive dressings may lead to skin maceration, to which the elderly are particularly vulnerable due to their aged skin (Cutting and White, 2002).

Baranoski (2001), Cuzzell (1990), and Murray (2005) all concur that one aim of treatment should be to prevent further trauma to the wound area and, if viable, to use the skin flap as the dressing itself. If the skin flap has rolled, or folded into itself, it should be gently unfolded/unrolled using moistened sterile gloves, forceps, or moistened cotton buds, and any residual blood clots should gently be irrigated away using either warm saline or tap water. It may be easier and more comfortable for the patient to do this with the wound area submerged, this is necessary when a limb is wounded (Valente *et al*, 2003). Any necrotic edges of the skin flap should be debrided, and the flap laid into position without any undue tension. It is important not to try and appose the skin flap with the wound edges. This is unlikely to succeed and may cause tension on the skin flap, resulting in necrosis. Similarly, if the flap is sutured, this may lead to necrosis due to tension (Sutton and Pritty, 1985; *Figure 3.1*). The skin flap may adhere, but if it does not, the wound has still been covered by skin, the most appropriate dressing.

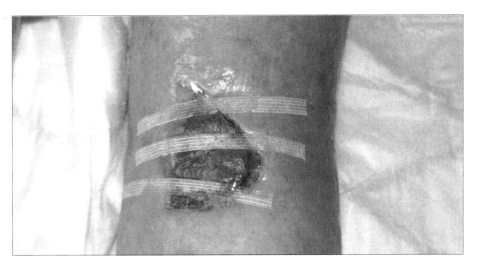

Figure 3.1: Necrosed skin flap. Skin tapes applied under tension

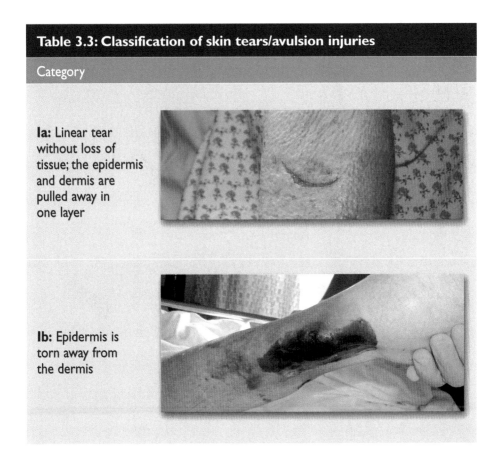

Table 3.3: Classification of skin tears/avulsion injuries

Category

Ia: Linear tear without loss of tissue; the epidermis and dermis are pulled away in one layer

Ib: Epidermis is torn away from the dermis

Table 3.3: Cont.

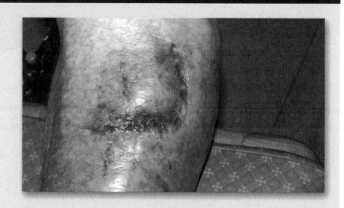

IIa: Skin tear with minimal or 25% or less loss of epidermis and dermis

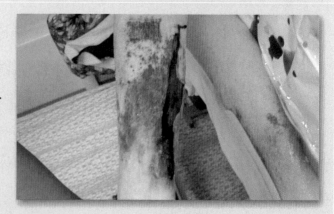

IIb: Skin tear with moderate or greater than 25% loss of epidermis and dermis

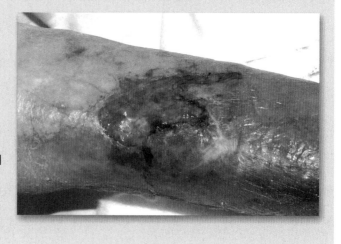

III: Skin tear with complete loss of epidermal tissue, caused by either initial trauma or infection. May also be partial-full dermal tissue loss

Not only is it vital to select the appropriate wound dressing (based on the wound bed, resulting exudate, and the surrounding skin), but also the individual patient and their ability to participate in their care must be considered. If the patient is confused or has dementia, they may remove dressings, possibly causing further trauma. A non-adherent dressing may be the most appropriate, regardless of the wound bed assessment. The vast majority of the elderly infirm with skin trauma are cared for either in hospital, a residential or nursing home, or by their practice nurse, and there may be discrepancy of knowledge between practitioners. Guidelines are necessary to enable the healthcare practitioner to treat skin tears appropriately and make an informed choice for their individual patient (Stephen-Haynes and Downing, 2003) (*Figure 3.2*).

Pre-tibial lacerations

Pre-tibial lacerations are commonly seen in A&E departments. This area of the body is particularly vulnerable as there is little soft tissue to provide protection. The pre-tibial area receives its blood supply in a longitudinal pattern from the perforators of the popliteal, peroneal and anterior tibial arteries, as such it is one of the areas of the body which has a reduced dermal blood supply (Pasyk *et al*, 1989).

Elderly individuals injure themselves by falling or knocking their legs against furniture, or other hard objects, and sustain a classical 'V-shaped' laceration (*Figure 3.3*). Dunkin *et al* (2003) proposed a classification for pre-tibial injuries (*Table 3.4*), together with an algorithm for their management. The classification is similar to the Payne, Martin (1993) classification for skin tears, but includes major degloving injuries. Dunkin *et al* (2003) also include guidance on mobilisation but, interestingly, concentrate predominantly on the medical management of pre-tibial injuries, not on the patient's wound management. While this might be useful to a medical practitioner, it has limited value to the nurse. To help communication between the patient and the healthcare professional involved in the management of a pre-tibial injury, an adaptation of the Dunkin *et al* (2003) algorithm may be helpful (*Figure 3.4*).

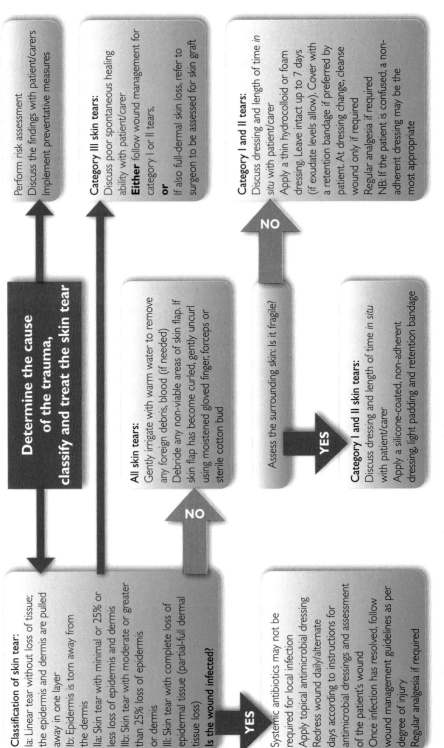

Classification of skin tear:
Ia: Linear tear without loss of tissue; the epidermis and dermis are pulled away in one layer
Ib: Epidermis is torn away from the dermis
IIa: Skin tear with minimal or 25% or less loss of epidermis and dermis
IIb: Skin tear with moderate or greater than 25% loss of epidermis or dermis
III: Skin tear with complete loss of epidermal tissue (partial-full dermal tissue loss)
Is the wound infected?

YES

Systemic antibiotics may not be required for local infection
Apply topical antimicrobial dressing
Redress wound daily/alternate days according to instructions for antimicrobial dressings and assessment of the patient's wound
Once infection has resolved, follow wound management guidelines as per degree of injury
Regular analgesia if required

Determine the cause of the trauma, classify and treat the skin tear

NO

All skin tears:
Gently irrigate with warm water to remove any foreign debris, blood (if needed)
Debride any non-viable areas of skin flap. If skin flap has become curled, gently uncurl using moistened gloved finger, forceps or sterile cotton bud

Assess the surrounding skin: Is it fragile?

YES

Category I and II skin tears:
Discuss dressing and length of time *in situ* with patient/carer
Apply a silicone-coated, non-adherent dressing, light padding and retention bandage

NO

Perform risk assessment
Discuss the findings with patient/carers
Implement preventative measures

Category III skin tears:
Discuss poor spontaneous healing ability with patient/carer
Either follow wound management for category I or II tears,
or
If also full-dermal skin loss, refer to surgeon to be assessed for skin graft

Category I and II tears:
Discuss dressing and length of time in situ with patient/carer
Apply a thin hydrocolloid or foam dressing. Leave intact up to 7 days (if exudate levels allow). Cover with a retention bandage if preferred by patient. At dressing change, cleanse wound only if required
Regular analgesia if required
NB: If the patient is confused, a non-adherent dressing may be the most appropriate

Figure 3.2: Skin tear assessment and treatment guideline

Table 3.4: Classification of pre-tibial injuries

Type I	Laceration
Type II	Laceration of flap with minimal haematoma and/or skin edge necrosis
Type III	Laceration of flap with moderate to severe haematoma and/or necrosis
Type IV	Major degloving injury

Much of the management of pre-tibial injuries has concentrated on the reconstruction problem for the medical practitioner, ie. the debate over whether or not to suture a skin flap (Sutton and Pritty, 1985). A survey of A&E departments in one region (Davis *et al*, 2004) highlighted a range of treatments for pre-tibial injuries: of 22 departments, 19 routinely used adhesive skin closures to close the wounds, but 3 departments sutured wounds. All wounds received additional dressings which ranged from paraffin gauze, silicone-coated dressings, saline-soaked gauze, and almost a third of departments used dry dressings. While all departments had a protocol for dealing with pre-tibial injuries, this varied, and few referred to a plastic surgeon, even when a plastic surgery department was on site. This study demonstrated a need for a consensus on treatments. Literature on the treatment of pre-tibial injuries suggests that suturing should be avoided and early skin grafting of severe injuries, types III and IV, helps to reduce healing times and, consequently, reduces the risk of infection and period of immobility due to injury (Haiart *et al*, 1990).

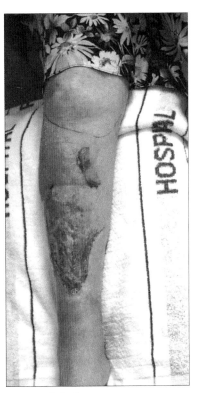

Figure 3.3: Large, characteristic 'V-shaped' pre-tibial laceration

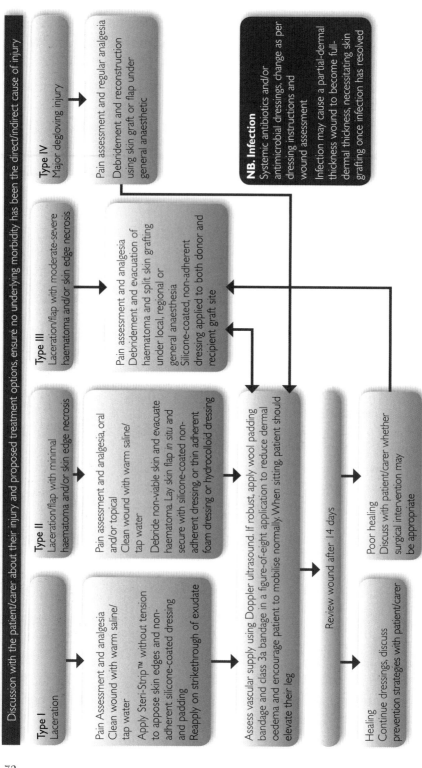

Figure 3.4: Algorithm for the management of pre-tibial injuries. Adapted from Dunkin *et al*, 2003

Bradley (2001) examined the treatment options for pre-tibial injuries in the older patient and concluded that assessment of the patient should include:

- cause and time of the injury
- any disease or medications which could delay healing
- the surface area of the wound, depth of the injury (facial damage or exposed tendon/periosteum), and viability of the skin flap.

The ability of the patient to participate in their own care must also be assessed and may influence treatment options.

The above factors determine management choices: whether conservative treatment using wound dressings and supportive light compression bandaging, or early surgical intervention via debridement, evacuation of haematoma and skin grafting is appropriate. Compression bandaging of a limb must be preceded by Doppler assessment to exclude underlying arterial disease. However, compression bandaging has been shown to be effective in improving the arterial blood flow in the lower limb (Mayrovitz *et al*, 1997; Mayrovitz, 1998), possibly by reducing dermal oedema leading to an improved dermal capillary flow with consequent improved healing ability. Bradley (2001) concludes that risk assessment is vital to identify the cause and circumstances of the injury, coupled with appropriate patient/carer education for prevention of further injury.

Skin trauma caused by wound dressings

Trauma to the skin may be caused by wound dressing adhesives, resulting in the epidermis being torn away with the skin, or by allergic contact dermatitis (ACD). The elderly have an increased propensity for ACD due to disruption of the immune response (Smith, 1989). ACD is often seen in the elderly with venous leg ulceration because of allergies to thiuram (a rubber accelerator), dyes, colophony, etc (Tavadia *et al*, 2003). Prior to selection of a wound dressing, the practitioner needs to assess not only the wound bed, but also the integrity of the surrounding skin to prevent further trauma. All factors must be considered and should influence dressing selection.

Skin assessment should include:

* ❖ *Colour:* is there evidence of senile purpura caused by dermal capillary vessels becoming thinner and more fragile, leading to the appearance of haemorrhage (White *et al*, 1994)?
* ❖ *Fragility:* is the skin smooth or wrinkled?
* ❖ *Texture:* is the skin robust and well-hydrated, or does it have a dry, papery appearance?
* ❖ *Oedema:* is this present, caused by local injury or systemic problems?
* ❖ *Scarring:* is there evidence of previous minor skin trauma?
* ❖ *Moisture:* is this present, due to perspiration, incontinence or wound exudate?
* ❖ *History:* is there any history of allergic contact dermatitis?

Wound exudate as a cause of skin trauma

Wound exudate, if not controlled by the use of absorbent dressings, may cause skin maceration. However, there are a vast range of absorbent dressings available, and not all perform in the same manner, or are available in the sizes and shapes which practitioners prefer (Hampton and Stephen-Haynes, 2005). Exudate management is dependent upon the ability of the practitioner to select an appropriate dressing which is not only the correct size, but is also able to absorb exudate and permit moisture evaporation (Grocott, 1998). The practitioner should also continually reassess the patient's wound to ensure that the dressing is changed frequently enough. If a dressing becomes completely saturated with exudate it will no longer perform as required, leading to excess moisture and possible breakdown of the peri-wound skin and enlargement of the wound (Cutting and White, 2002).

Maceration of the skin is caused by prolonged exposure to excess moisture and is seen as a complication in the management of many wound aetiologies, such as; pressure ulcers, leg ulcers, diabetic foot ulcers, fungating wounds, donor sites, fistulae and also the skin around percutaneous enterostomal gastrostomy (PEG) sites and stomas.

Maceration of the skin can affect all ages, but is more common in the pre-term neonate and the elderly due to their increased vulnerability. In pre-term neonatal skin there is an absence of subcutaneous tissue (Hardman, 2006), and so the skin lies directly on muscle, causing its red appearance. The high rate of transepidermal water loss leads to a moist skin surface which, in turn, substantially increases the potential for skin damage (Rutter, 1996). Nasogastric tubes or nasal cannulae may also be *in situ*, thus increasing the risk of friction injuries, which highlights the need to continuously monitor the pre-term neonate.

In the elderly, excessive moisture leads to rapid deterioration of the skin due to thinning of the dermis and reduction of subcutaneous tissue, rendering the skin vulnerable to maceration. This is frequently seen at the sacral area when urinary incontinence is not well-managed and the skin becomes more permeable, increasing the risk of infection. Similarly, wet wound areas increase the skin's permeability, and maceration occurs more easily than in the younger adult. It is vital to consider the age and the skin of the individual in wound management.

Conclusion

Skin trauma is easily sustained at each end of the age spectrum, the very young and the very old. This increased propensity for trauma is directly related to the immature state of the skin in the pre-term neonate, and the impaired structure of the skin in the elderly. When dealing with patients in these at-risk groups, it is essential that a risk assessment of the skin be undertaken, together with appropriate measures to prevent skin trauma. From the management of existing trauma there is now increasing evidence from clinical research that there are guidelines, dressings and patient-centred considerations leading to optimal treatment. It is no longer acceptable that an *ad hoc* approach is taken to the management of skin trauma in these groups.

References

Baranoski S (2000) Skin tears: staying on guard against the enemy of frail skin. *Nursing* **30**(9): 41–7

Baranoski S (2001) Skin tears: Guard against this enemy of frail skin. *Nurs Management* **32**(8): 25–32

Bradley L (2001) Pre-tibial lacerations in older patients: the treatment options. *J Wound Care* **10**(1): 521–3

Braverman IM, Fonferko E (1982) Studies in cutaneous aging II The microvasculature. *J Invest Dermatol* **78**: 444–8

Butcher M, White R (2005) The structure and functions of the skin. In: White R, ed. *Skin Care and Wound Management: Assessment, management and treatment.* Wounds UK, Aberdeen

Camp-Sorrell D (1991) Skin tears: what can you do? *Oncol Nurs Forum* **18**(1): 135

Cutting KF, White RJ (2002) Maceration of the skin and wound bed: 1: The nature and causes of maceration. *J Wound Care* **11**(7): 275–8

Cuzzell JZ (1990) Clues: bruised, torn skin. *Am J Nurs* **18**: 16–18

Cuzzell JZ (2002) Wound assessment and evaluation: Skin tear protocol. *Dermatol Nurs* **14**(6): 405

Davis A, Chester D, Allison K, Davison P (2004) A Survey of how a region's A&E units manage pre-tibial lacerations. *J Wound Care* **13**(1): 5–7

Department of Health (2004) Office for National Statistics, 2004. DoH, London. Available online at: www.dh.gov.uk/PublicationsandStatistics/ StatisticalWorkAreas/StatisiticalHealthcare/StatisticalHealthCareArticle/ fs/en

Dunkin CS, Elfleet D, Ling C, Brown TP (2003) A step-by-step guide to classifying and managing pretibial injuries. *J Wound Care* **12**(3): 109–11

Edwards H, Gaskill D, Nash R (1998) Treating skin tears in nursing home residents: A pilot study comparing four types of dressings. *Int J Nurs Practice* **4**(1): 25–32

Fenske NA, Conard CB (1988) Aging skin. *Am Fam Phys* **37**(2): 219–30

Foster KG, Ellis FP, Dore C, Exton-Smith AN, Weiner JS (1976) Sweat responses in the aged. *Age Ageing* **5**: 91–101

Gilchrist BA, Murphy GF, Sorter NA (1982) Effect of chronologic aging and ultraviolet irradiation on Langerhans cells in human epidermis. *J Invest Dermatol* **79**: 85–8.

Grocott P (1998) Exudate management in fungating wounds. *J Wound Care* **7**(9): 445–8

Grove GL (1986) Physiologic changes in older skin. *Dermatologic Clin* **4**(3): 425–32

Gurwitz JH, Sanchez-Cross MT, Eckler MA, Matulis J (1994) The epidemiology of adverse and unexpected events in the long-term care setting. *J Am Geriatr Soc* **42**(1): 33–8

Haiart DC, Paul AB, Chalmers R, Griffiths JMT (1990) Pretibial lacerations: a comparison of primary excision and grafting with 'defatting' the flap. *Br J Plast Surg* **43**: 312–14

Hamilton S (2004) Caring for the skin of older residents: a practical guide. *Nurs Residential Care* **6**(7): 326–9

Hampton S, Stephen-Haynes J (2005) Skin maceration: assessment, prevention and treatment. In: White R, ed. _Skin Care in Wound Management: Assessment, prevention and treatment._ Wounds UK, Aberdeen

Hardman M (2006) In utero skin development. In: Denyer J, White R, eds. _Paediatric Skin and Wound Care._ Wounds UK, Aberdeen

Lavker RM (1979) Structural alterations in exposed and unexposed aged skin. _J Invest Dermatol_ 73: 59–66

Mayrovitz HN, Delgado M, Smith J (1997) Compression bandaging effects on lower extremity peripheral and subbandage skin blood perfusion. _Wounds_ 9(5): 146–52

Mayrovitz HN (1998) Compression-induced pulsatile blood flow in human legs. _Clin Physiol_ 18(2): 117–24

Meuleneire F (2002) Using a soft silicone-coated net dressing to manage skin tears. _J Wound Care_ 11(10): 365–9

Montagna W, Carlisle K (1979) Structural changes in aging human skin. _J Investe Dermatol_ 73: 47–53

Murray E (2005) Guidelines for the management of skin tears. St Vincents & Mater Health; Sydney Nursing Monograph. Available online at: www.clininfo.health.nsw.gov.au/hospolic/stvincents/index

Nazarko L (2005) Preventing and treating skin tears. _Nurs Residential Care_ 7(12): 549–50

Nursing and Midwifery Council (2004) _The NMC Code of Professional Conduct: standards for conduct, performance and ethics._ NMC, London. Available online at: www.nmc-uk.org

Payne RL, Martin MC (1993) Defining and classifying skin tears: Need for a common language. _Ostomy/Wound Management_ 39(5): 16–20, 22–24, 26

Pasyk KA, Thomas SV, Hassett CA, Cherry GW, Faller R (1989) Regional differences in capillary density of the normal human dermis. _Plast Reconstr Surg_ 83(6): 939–45

Penzer R, Finch M (2001) Promoting healthy skin in older people. _Nurs Standard_ 15: 46–52

Pichard C, Kyle UG, Morabier A, Perrier A, Vermeulan B, Unger P (2004) Nutritional Assessment: lean body mass depletion at hospital admission is associated with an increased length of stay. _Am J Clin Nutrition_ 79(4): 613–18

Procacci P, Bozza G, Buzzelli G, Della Corte M (1970) The cutaneous pricking pain threshold in old age. _Gerontologica Clinico_ 12: 213–18

Richey ML, Richey HK, Fenske NA (1988) Aging-related skin changes: Development and clinical meaning. _Geriatrics_ 43(4): 49–64

Rutter N (1996) The immature skin. _Eur J Pediatr_ 155(suppl 2): S18–S20

Shuster S, Black MM, McVitie E (1975) The influence of age and sex on skin thickness, skin collagen and density. *Br J Dermatol* **93**: 639–43

Smith L (1989) Histopathologic characteristics and ultrastructure of aging skin. *Cutis* **43**: 414–24

Solomon LM, Virtue C (1975) The biology of cutaneous aging. *Int J Dermatol* **14**: 172–81

Stephen-Haynes J, Downing P (2003) The development and implementation of an acute, traumatic guideline. *Br J Community Nurs* (Wound Care Supplement) **8**(3): 8–16

Stout NR, Kenny RA, Bayliss PH (1999) A review of the water balance in ageing in health and disease. *Gerontology* **45**(2): 61–7

Sutton R, Pritty P (1985) Use of sutures or adhesive tapes for primary closure of pre-tibial lacerations. *Br Med J* **290**(6482): 1627

Tavadia S, Bianchi J, Dawe RS, McEvoy M, Wiggens E, Hamill E *et al* (2003) Allergic contact dermatitis in venous leg ulcer patients. *Contact Dermatitis* **48**: 261–5

Thomas DR, Goode PS, La Master K, Tennyson T, Parnell LK (1999) A comparison of an opaque foam dressing versus a transparent film dressing in the management of skin tears in institutional subjects. *Ostomy/Wound Management* **45**: 22–4, 27–8

Thomas S (2003) Atraumatic dressings. Available online at: <u>www.worldwidewounds.com/2003/january/thomas/Atraumatic-Dressings</u>

Valente JH, Forti RJ, Freundlich LF, Zandieh SO, Crane EF (2003) Wound Irrigation in Children. *Ann Emerg Med* **41**(5): 609–16

White MW, Karam S, Cowell B (1994) Skin tears in frail elders: a practical approach to prevention. *Geriatr Nurs* **15**(2): 95–9

CHAPTER 4

WOUND PAIN AND DRESSINGS

Deborah Hofman

Patients with chronic wounds are likely to be in pain and, for many patients, the worst aspect of their wound is the pain that it causes, rather than other aspects which affect quality of life such as exudate, odour, and restricted mobility. The presence of unrelieved pain is likely to delay healing, leading to a vicious circle of pain, emotional debilitation, poor concordance, and slow healing (*Figure 4.1*).

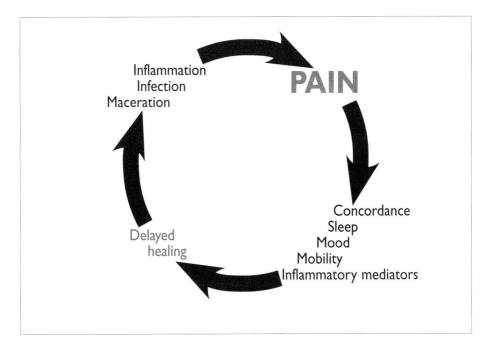

Figure 4.1: Vicious circle of pain

It has become widely recognised that the problem of pain associated with chronic wounds is often ignored and/or poorly managed, resulting in prolonged suffering (Dallam, 1995; Hofman, 1997; Noonan and Burge, 1998; Moffatt, 2002). Persistent pain is often marginalised or ignored because it can be a difficult problem to resolve. Moreover, older patients with chronic wounds are often reluctant to take medication, either because they are already on multiple medicines, or because they are concerned about the side-effects, eg. confusion, constipation, nausea and nightmares. If there are ways of managing wound pain that can reduce the need for systemic analgesia, they should be considered. Over the last decade, industry and wound care practitioners have been paying more attention to the role of dressings in reducing wound pain (Thomas, 1994; Dallam *et al*, 1995; Briggs, 1996; Hofman and Cooper, 2005; Hollinworth, 2005).

This chapter concentrates on leg ulceration, although much of what is discussed is relevant to other types of chronic wounds where pain is a problem.

Wound assessment

Before considering dressing choice for a patient, a full assessment should be undertaken to determine the aetiology of the wound and the possible cause(s) of wound pain. In many cases, a dressing will not enhance healing or relieve pain. It is important to establish the cause of a wound to instigate correct treatment which may, of itself, bring pain relief. The practitioner must be clear as to what is causing the ulcer in addition to what is causing the pain.

Leg ulceration assessment is a complex process and with an increasingly elderly and frail population it is common to see multiple pathologies. An accurate diagnosis must be established, although it may be necessary to address the problem of pain in the first instance. This may mean systemic analgesia, soothing dressings, and withholding compression (if indicated) until the pain has been resolved. All leg ulcers may be painful, and the pain may result from one or more causes. For example, leg pain may be related to the damage to the surrounding skin or underlying vascular structures, or arise from the wound itself. Patients may also have underlying arthritic and/or muscle pain. In addition, there may well be an emotional component

(*Table 4.1*). Not all types of pain are amenable to relief by dressings alone and a multidisciplinary approach is required.

Dressings are helpful in controlling pain in the skin and at the wound site, and are also beneficial in patients suffering from hypersensitivity and wind-up pain (*Chapter 2*). However, dressings are unlikely to have any beneficial effect on some of the other causes of pain listed in *Table 4.1*, eg. allodynia, phlebitis, arthritis, or claudication. Involving the patient in dressing choice and dressing removal may help to reduce the negative psychological aspects.

Table 4.1: Leg ulcer pain	
Skin	Maceration, dermatitis, infection, inflammation, oedema, lipodermatosclerosis, atrophie blanche
Vascular	Phlebitis, ischaemia, deep vein thrombosis (DVT)
Muscular	Cramp, claudication
Skeletal	Arthritis, gout
Nerve	Neuropathy (allodynia, hypersensitivity, wind-up)
Wound	Infection, inflammation, injury, poor exudate management
Psychological	Depression, anger, fear

Useful pain

Pain is the body's alarm signal for tissue damage and, therefore, pain assessment should be given the same priority as assessment of temperature, pulse, respiration and blood pressure, and should be regarded as the fifth vital sign (Turk and Melzack, 2001). In wounds, tissue damage may be caused by infection, inflammation, or ischaemia. It may also be iatrogenic, being caused by bandaging or inappropriate dressings. It is necessary to establish the cause of the pain before considering dressing choice (*Table 4.2*).

Table 4.2: Useful pain (the four Is)	
Causes of pain	Dressings/treatments to consider
Infection	• systemic antibiotics • antimicrobial dressings (iodine, silver, honey dressings – iodine and honey may cause increased pain – and metronidazole gel) • antibiotic creams
Inflammation	• new generation hydrogels • topical anti-inflammatory treatment
Ischaemia	• check Doppler reading (refer to vascular unit if appropriate) • avoid pressure on area • choose dressings that promote angiogenesis, eg. hydrocolloids, lipidocolloids, second-generation hydrogels
Iatrogenic	• check dressings and bandaging are not causing tissue damage • allow more time at dressing change • consider analgesia prior to dressing change and/ or Entonox® • consider patch testing

Infection

High bacterial load will increase pain levels even before frank infection is apparent. Wound infection without cellulitis can also be identified by signs such as change of granulation tissue, increased exudate and odour, as well as an increase of pain. Many patients report immediate pain relief when systemic antibiotics are prescribed, even when there are no signs of cellulitis. It would, therefore, be reasonable to suppose that dressings which reduce the bacterial bioburden of the wound will also relieve pain. Unfortunately, some of these dressings can cause increased pain on application (eg. iodine and honey dressings).

For the last ten to fifteen years, most topical antimicrobials have been out of vogue with wound care practitioners, although cadexomer iodine dressings have retained a role, especially with the emergence of *methicillin-resistant Staphylococcus aureus* (MRSA). However, iodine dressings may be painful and many patients cannot tolerate them.

Honey dressings have recently become popular in the management of heavily colonised/infected wounds (Cooper *et al*, 1999; Cooper and Molan, 1999), although many patients report a drawing sensation when these dressings are applied. This can be intolerable so they are not the first choice for very painful wounds (Hollinworth, 2005). Nevertheless, there is a honey dressing with a lower honey content which, reportedly, causes less pain and is suitable for sensitive wounds. In the author's experience, silver sulfadiazine cream (SSD cream) is often soothing on painful wounds, but it is unclear whether this is because it is a cool cream or because its antibacterial action is analgesic. SSD cream can be used in conjunction with a non-adherent or soft silicone dressing, but is not appropriate in heavily exuding wounds. A lipidocolloid impregnated with silver sulfadiazine is available, which is useful in managing wet wounds where application of a cream is not appropriate (Carsin *et al*, 2004). *Pseudomonas* thrives in wet wounds and causes increased exudate, maceration, and soreness of the surrounding skin, as well as producing proteases which trigger inflammation and pain (see below).

Over the last few years, there has been much interest in the role of dressings containing silver in the management of bacteria (Thomas, 2003; Bowler, 2004; Lansdown, 2005). Absorbent silver dressings have been developed which absorb exudate as well as releasing silver into the wound. These are particularly beneficial in wet, heavily colonised wounds. Dressings which hold exudate next to the skin increase skin damage and pain and this is true of some foam dressings (*Figure 4.2*). Dressings which draw exudate away from the skin surface should, therefore, be selected. Chronic wounds are often heavily colonised with anaerobic bacteria which can be treated by metronidazole gel. Caution, however, should be used in patients taking warfarin as metronidazole enhances the anticoagulant effect.

Wounds where there is necrotic tissue or slough will have a heavy bioburden (Bellingeri and Hofman, 2006), and consequent inflammation and pain. Once the necrotic tissue is removed the wound may be less painful, although the process itself, be it sharp debridement or larval therapy, may cause pain. Topical anaesthesia is effective when applied to the wound prior to sharp debridement, although it is not licensed for this purpose (Hansson *et al*, 1993). Moist dressings which enhance autolysis are a gentler approach than sharp debridement, although the process will take longer. However, new generation hydrogel sheets appear to have a much faster debriding action than hydrogels (Armitage and Roberts, 2004).

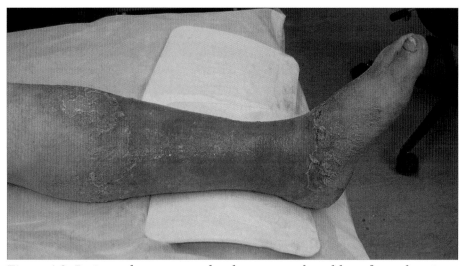

Figure 4.2: Patient whose eczema has been exacerbated by a foam dressing keeping exudate in contact with the skin

Inflammation

Chronic inflammation in the wound is considered to be one of the major factors in delayed healing (Agren *et al*, 2000). The inflammatory mediators that modulate wound healing can also induce pain by triggering nociceptors, and add to the heightened perception of pain by lowering the triggering threshold of nociceptors (Cunha *et al*, 2005). Inflammation is associated with infection, but can be present in a wound that is otherwise showing no signs of infection (Agren *et al*, 2000). Inflammation would, therefore, appear to be an important feature of persistent pain in patients with chronic wounds. In wounds where inflammation is a problem, there is a growing interest in some specialist centres in the role of topical corticosteroids, but their use remains controversial and they should not be applied by the non-specialist as there are increased risks of infection, contact sensitivity, and reduced vascularisation of the wound. Dressings which have been impregnated with non-steroidal anti-inflammatory agents may prove a useful tool in the management of the painful wound. Clinical experience has shown that new generation hydrogel sheets, which appear to reduce inflammation, are beneficial in the management of persistent wound pain (Armitage and Roberts, 2004).

A wound that is inflamed will be sensitive and non-adhesive silicone dressings may be helpful. Such dressings have also been shown to be invaluable in the management of patients with wounds associated with auto-immune disorders, such as systemic lupus erythematosus or scleroderma, where the surrounding skin tends to be painful, as well as in the management of children with hereditary fragile skin (epidemolysis bullosa). Adhesive soft silicone dressings have proved especially useful on fragile/tender skin.

Ischaemia

Patients with ischaemic wounds should, where appropriate, be reviewed by a vascular surgeon. In some cases, little can be done surgically to enhance the vascularisation of the wound. In others, the large vessels may be adequate (normal ankle brachial pressure index [ABPI]), but the microcirculation is impaired, eg. in patients with diabetes, patients who smoke, or in patients with microcirculatory disorders, such as sickle cell anaemia, Raynaud's phenomenon). These wounds are normally very painful. Dressings which keep the wound moist and encourage angiogenesis may help to relieve the pain, such as soft silicone dressings, hydrocolloids, hydrogels, and hydrogel sheets.

Iatrogenic-induced pain

All too often, it is the person changing the dressing who causes or exacerbates pain. Pain at dressing change is sometimes difficult to avoid and has been extensively covered in two consensus documents (European Wound Management Association [EWMA], 2002; World Union of Wound Healing Societies [WUWHS], 2004). Most of us can identify with a patient's fear at dressing pain having had our own childhood experience of dressings being painfully removed. We have, it is to be hoped, moved on since William Henley wrote a poem entitled, 'Waiting', of his experiences of having a tuberculous wound dressed at the end of the nineteenth century:

Angry and sore I wait to be admitted
Wait till my heart is lead upon my stomach

While at their ease two dressers do their chores
One has a probe — it feels to me a crow bar...

The poet clearly illustrates how pain is exacerbated by his anger, fear, and resentment. Clinicians can do much to alleviate pain by addressing these emotions in patients.

When pain at dressing change is anticipated to be severe, or when the patient is afraid of potential pain, systemic analgesia or Entonox® (50% nitrous oxide and 50% oxygen gas) may be given.

However, in most cases, selection of a genuinely non-adherent dressing is sufficient. Where there is insufficient exudate, alginates or cellulose dressings will adhere and be difficult to remove. Hydrogels with a non-adherent dressing and pad may also adhere badly (*Figure 4.3*). Traditional dressings, such as gauze and paraffin gauze, often cause trauma and pain on removal and should be avoided (WUWHS, 2004). More modern, adhesive-backed dressings can also cause trauma to fragile skin around the wound and to the wound bed (Hollinworth, 2005); whereas soft silicone or lipidocolloid dressings do not adhere to the wound bed or surrounding skin, and can remain in place for several days so that only the cover dressing is removed. This is of great benefit to a patient who has come to dread dressing changes.

If a patient complains of increased pain following dressing application or bandaging, it may be an indication of tissue injury and the dressing should be removed and the wound re-assessed. The problem of contact sensitivity, and the implications of applying a dressing to which the patient has become sensitised, is dealt with in *Chapter 6*.

Applying a moist dressing to a heavily exudating wound will increase pain and tissue damage. Although it is well-established that a moist environment enhances epithelialisation (Bishop *et al*, 2003), it is also the case that wound exudate is a corrosive biological fluid rich in enzymes which destroys epithelial cells and causes maceration of the surrounding skin (Trengrove *et al*, 1999; Cutting and White, 2002). Moisture balance is crucial not only for patient comfort, but also to provide a good healing environment. The practitioner must become expert at assessing exudate quantity and in choosing dressings which will hydrate, but not over-hydrate a wound, as well as absorbing excess exudate.

Bandage injury is unfortunately common and, in a patient with normal sensation, will be preceded by pain. A patient should always be asked whether he is comfortable with the dressing and bandage applied. Nurses should anticipate problems in cases where ulceration occurs over bony prominences, or in sites where bandage creasing will exacerbate a wound (*Figure 4.4*). Cushioning dressings, such as hydrocolloids or foams, can reduce pressure and tissue injury.

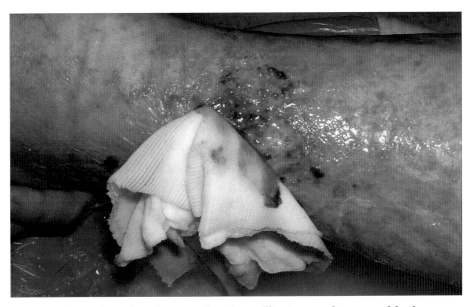

Figure 4.3: Hydrogel and gauze dressing adhering to the wound bed, causing pain and trauma on removal

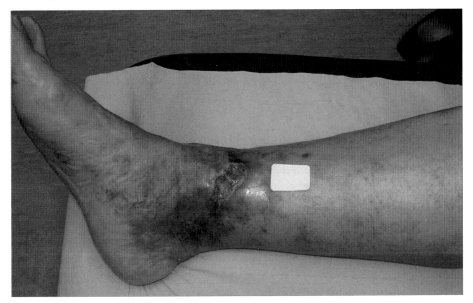

Figure 4.4: Venous ulcer where compression bandage caused increased pain and trauma. Resolved by a hydrocolloid dressing and compression hosiery

Useless pain

Pain caused by damaged nerves (neuropathic pain) performs no useful function in terms of prevention of tissue damage, but can be severely debilitating for the patient.

Neuropathic pain

Careful assessment of wound pain will enable an alert practitioner to identify neuropathic pain, which is common in patients with long-standing wounds. Some neuropathic pain has a different quality from nociceptive pain and is often described as shooting, burning, stabbing or electric shock-like in quality (Cooper and Hofman, 2003). Patients may experience allodynia, where the wound is more or less insensate but the adjacent tissues are hypersensitive and even stroking is unbearable, or hyperalgesia, where the wound has become over a period of time exquisitely painful, and the lightest touch is unbearable. Wind-up pain, associated with long-standing tissue damage, results in an increase in the perceived intensity of pain. Neuropathic pain normally responds well to oral medication (*Chapter 8*), but dressing choice also has an important part to play. Patients with neuropathic pain will often benefit from a completely non-adherent dressing (eg. a soft silicone or lipidocolloid dressing). In the case of patients suffering from hyperalgesia, a soothing dressing such as a hydrogel or hydrogel sheet may be beneficial. In cases of severe persistent pain, topical morphine or diamorphine mixed with a hydrogel has been shown to be beneficial (Back and Finlay, 1995; Twillman *et al*, 1999; Grocott, 2000; Ashfield, 2005). Topical application, as opposed to systemic administration, has the advantage of minimising the side-effects of opioids (Ashfield, 2005). Patients suffering from wind-up pain or hyperalgesia will need extra care and time during dressing and wound interventions, to allow for reassurance and ensure good communication between the patient and practitioner. It is important to educate practitioners dealing with patients suffering from these types of pain, so that the unusual sensations that these patients report are clearly understood and not dismissed.

Conclusion

There are as yet no randomised control trials (RCTs) listed in the Cochrane database that prove that any dressing has superior pain-relieving qualities over another. However, there is a wealth of expert evidence in the form of published case studies, which can guide practitioners dealing with painful wounds to make sensible and informed choices. The ultimate choice should, of course, rest with the patient who, alone, can make a pronouncement on the pain — relieving qualities or comfort of a dressing. What works for one patient may well not work for another. The best qualities a practitioner working in the field of wound care can have are to listen intelligently, and to use experience and knowledge effectively to make informed choices in the attempt to alleviate persistent wound pain and promote healing.

References

Agren MS, Eaglstein WH, Ferguson MW, Harding KG, Moore K, Saarialhokere UK, Schultz GS (2000) Causes and effects of the chronic inflammation in venous leg ulcers. *Acta Derm Venereol Suppl* (Stock) **210**: 3–17

Armitage M, Roberts J (2004) Caring for patients with leg ulcers and an underlying vasculitic condition. *Br J Community Nurs* Dec Suppl: S16–S21

Ashfield T (2005) The use of topical opioids to relieve pressure ulcer pain. *Nurs Standard* **19**(45): 90–2

Back IN, Finlay I (1995) Analgesic effect of topical opioids on painful skin ulcers. *J Pain Symptom Manage* **10**(7): 493

Bellingeri A, Hofman D (2006) Debridement of pressure ulcers. In: Romanelli M, Clark M, Cherry G, Colin D, Defloor T, eds. *Science Practice of Pressure Ulcer Management*. Springer, London: 131

Bishop SM, Walker M, Rogers AA, Chen WY (2003) Importance of moisture balance at the wound dressing interface. *J Wound Care* **12**(4): 125–8

Briggs M (1996) Surgical wound pain: a trial of two treatments. *J Wound Care* **5**(10): 456–60

Bowler PG (2004) Infection: the role of bacterial communities in wound healing. Paper presented at 2nd World Union of Wound Healing Societies meeting, Paris

Carsin H, Wasserman D, Pannier M, Dumas R, Bohbot S (2004) A silver sulphadiazine-impregnated lipidocolloid wound dressing to treat second-degree burns. *J Wound Care* 13(4): 145–8

Cooper S, Hofman D (2003) Leg ulcers and pain: A review. *Int J Lower Extremity Wounds* 2(4): 198–207

Cooper RA, Molan PC (1999) The use of honey as an antiseptic in managing Pseudomonas infection. *J Wound Care* 8(4): 161–4

Cooper RA, Molan PC, Harding KG (1999) Antibacterial activity of honey against strains of *Staphylococcus aureus* from infected wounds. *J R Soc Med* 92: 283–5

Cunha TM, Verri WA, Silva JS *et al* (2005) A cascade of cytokines mediates mechanical inflammatory hypernociception in mice. *PNAS* 102(5): 1755–60

Cutting KF, White RJ (2002) Maceration of the wound bed 1, its nature and causes. *J Wound Care* 11: 275–8

Dallam L, Smythe C *et al* (1995) Pressure ulcer pain: assessment and quantification. *JWOCN* 22(5): 211–17

European Wound Management Association (EWMA) (2002) *Position Document: Pain at wound dressing changes*. Medical Education Partnership Ltd, London

Grocott P (2000) The management of malignant wounds. *Eur J Palliative Nurs* 8(5): 214–21

Hansson C, Holm J, Lillieborg S, Syren A (1993) Repeated treatment with lidocaine/prilocaine cream (EMLA) as a topical anaesthetic for the cleansing of venous leg ulcers. *Acta Derma Venereal* (Stock) 73: 231–3

Hofman D, Lindholm C, Arnold F *et al* (1997) Pain in venous leg ulcers. *J Wound Care* 6: 222–4

Hofman D, Cooper S (2005) Towards understanding and managing pain in leg ulcers. *Dermatol Practice* 13(1): 10–12

Hollinworth H (2005) The management of patients' pain in wound care. *Nurs Standard* 20(7): 65–73

Lansdown ABG, Williams A *et al* (2005) Silver absorption and antibacterial efficacy of silver dressings. *J Wound Care* 14(4): 155–60

Moffatt CJ, Franks PJ, Hollinworth H (2002) Understanding wound pain and trauma: an international perspective. EWMA Position Document (2002) *Pain at Wound Dressing Changes*. Medical Education Partnership, London

Noonan L, Burge SM (1998) Venous leg ulcers: is pain a problem? *Phlebology* 13: 14–19

Thomas S (1994) Low-adherence dressings. *J Wound Care* 3(1): 27–30

Thomas S (2003) A comparison of the antimicrobial effects of four silver-containing dressings on three organisms. *J Wound Care* **12**(3): 101–7

Trengrove NJ, Stacey MC, MacAuley S *et al* (1999) Analysis of the acute and chronic wound environments: the role of proteases and their inhibitors. *Wound Rep Regen* 7: 442–52

Turk DC, Melzack R (2001) Preface. In: Turk D, Melzack R, eds. *Handbook of Pain Asssessment*. The Guildford Press, New York: viii

Twillman RK, Long TD, Cathers TA, Mueller DW (1999) Treatment of painful skin ulcers with topical opioids. *J Pain Symptom Manage* **17**(4): 288–92

World Union of Wound Healing Societies (2004) *Principles of Best Practice: Minimising pain at wound dressing-related procedures. A consensus document.* Medical Education Partnership Ltd, London. Available online at: www.wuwhs.org/pdf/consensus_eng.pdf

CHAPTER 5

ASSESSMENT OF WOUND PAIN AT DRESSING CHANGE

Marco Romanelli and Valentina Dini

The dressing change in a patient with either an acute or a chronic wound is always a difficult task and can be a major challenge for the caregiver. In daily practice, more and more often patients with chronic wounds are asking the clinician to treat and control the pain associated with their wounds, rather than expecting rapid and complete healing. Minimising trauma and pain at dressing change is becoming a vital area of wound care, and one that has been brought consistently to the attention of doctors and nurses over the last few years (mainly through the recognition that this topic had previously been underestimated when compared to healing as the principal aim of treatment). Since the first publication by Winter (1962) on the role of moist wound healing, one of the key elements when compared to dry dressings, has been the control of wound pain (Eaglstein, 1993). At that time, the better control of wound pain was explained by the soothing of nerve endings in a moist environment, and the prevention of dehydration of nerve receptors. However, today, we are aware of several more cellular and biochemical aspects to consider (Schultz *et al*, 2005).

This chapter covers the principles of best practice in minimising pain and trauma during wound dressing-related procedures by using the first European Wound Management Association (EWMA) position document (EWMA, 2002) and the World Union of Wound Healing Societies (WUWHS) consensus document (WUWHS, 2004).

Pain assessment at dressing change

Pain assessment in patients with cutaneous wounds is a comprehensive procedure, including all their daily activities, especially those requiring pharmacological treatment. However, less attention is given to the assessment of pain before, during and after individual dressing-related procedures (Reddy *et al*, 2003). Wound clinics are busy places and frequently the time devoted to each patient is not sufficient to address all the issues surrounding wound management. The different types of wounds and the individual patient responses affected by age, cultural and psychosocial aspects, mean that each pain assessment at dressing change should be individualised and documented in the patient's records to allow audit of outcomes to be performed. A 'pain diary' will provide the clinician and the patient with a useful tool to help correlate strategic treatment with different outcomes at specific times of the day.

Pain scales

Routine pain assessment can be undertaken using different pain scales, which are not suitable for all patients and must be adapted according to individual patient's needs and/or circumstances. The numerical (NRS) (*Figure 5.1*) and verbal (VRS) (*Figure 5.2*) rating scales are useful in patients with chronic wounds. The NRS provides the patient with a range of numbers from 0 to 10 indicating the range from 'no pain' to 'worst possible pain'. The patient is asked to choose a number on the scale according to his or her level of pain. The VRS is a simple scale which uses no more than four of five words to describe the intensity of the pain, such as: none, mild, moderate or severe. There are also visual scales which use cartoon faces ranging from a smiling face for 'no pain' to a tearful face for 'worst pain'. However, a practical and currently well-accepted way to perform pain assessment is by talking to the patients about their feelings and using a more integrated type of questioning, instead of the direct, short questions aimed at receiving only a concise 'yes' or 'no' answer. In particular, talking to an elderly patient about his or her pain during dressing-related procedures makes it easier to identify factors which may influence or aggravate this procedure, especially when done outside the control of wound care specialists. In a recent survey performed in France (Meaume *et al*, 2004) on the incidence of pain during dressing removal in patients with acute and chronic wounds, a severity score was used. In this study, dressing removal was the most painful procedure affecting 85% of patients with acute wounds, and cleansing was reported as frequently painful in 97% of patients with chronic wounds. The most painful dressing-related aspect of care was the adherence of dressings to the wound bed, which was reported respectively in 55% and 38% of acute and chronic wounds. Pain assessment at the time of a dressing-change procedure may be a good indicator of the appropriateness of the treatment chosen. During the procedure, the caregiver must deal with several aspects that can act as a trigger for wound pain. The condition of bandages, the modification of the wound dressing over time, and the appearance of the wound bed are key elements to be monitored in relation to pain assessment.

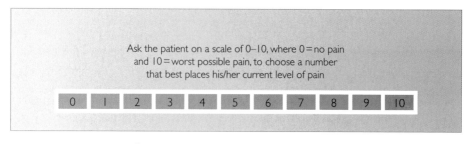

Figure 5.1: Numerical rating scale. Reproduced by kind permission of the World Union of Wound Healing Societies (WUWHS, 2004)

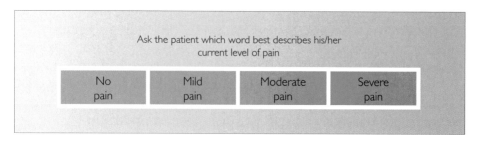

Figure 5.2: Verbal rating scale. Reproduced by kind permission of the World Union of Wound Healing Societies (WUWHS, 2004)

Pain in different wound types at dressing change

The intensity of pain may be quite different in chronic wounds of varying aetiologies which has to be considered in pain prevention and management strategies. Also, the dressing change-related procedure can vary slightly depending on the anatomical location of the wound, and the time required to perform the procedure.

Venous leg ulcers

In patients with venous leg ulcers, compared to other types of chronic wounds (Sibbald, 1998), there are several aspects which can aggravate dressing change-related procedures. Moisture balance is essential in venous leg ulcers, and an excessive amount of exudate can affect the dressing change, mainly because of the level of tissue damage on the surrounding skin, which can range from red to white maceration or include new areas of tissue breakdown. An increased amount of exudate is also a clinical sign of infection, and the bacterial balance must be kept constantly under control to prevent an increase in pain intensity during dressing change. Venous ulcers of the lower leg are often associated with dermatitis that affects the surrounding skin, with various degrees of skin desquamation, inflammation/erythema and pigmentation. At the time of a dressing change, the caregiver must pay careful attention to the condition of the wound bed and surrounding skin which may exacerbate the level of pain. The removal of a multilayer bandaging system is a critical procedure, which often increases the level of anxiety in patients who are afraid of further trauma during this process. Every effort must be made to keep this intervention under control by reassuring patients and making them as comfortable as possible. Pain assessment at dressing change must be systematically carried out to relate the various aspects of the procedure (bandaging, dressing removal, dressing application, etc) to the intensity of the pain (Hofman *et al*, 1997). See *Chapter 7*, 'Pain in venous leg ulcers and its impact on quality of life'.

Diabetic foot ulcers

Metabolic abnormalities in diabetes may lead to arterial disease and neuropathy. Foot ulcers represent a lower extremity complication in patients with diabetes (Lavery *et al*, 1998), although pain is uncommon in neuropathic foot ulcers because of damage to the sensory motor and autonomic fibres. The presence of pain in diabetic foot ulcers is mostly associated with deep infection (Caputo *et al*, 1997), or critical limb ischaemia (Frykberg, 2002). Surgical debridement is the treatment of choice when infection is likely to spread over the foot and lower leg, increasing the risk of amputation. At this time, the dressing change-related procedure is influenced by the use of various forms of offloading by clinicians. Local wound care should be in accordance with the principles of moist wound healing, but with more frequent dressing changes due to the high risk of infection and wound deterioration.

Pressure ulcers

Wound pain assessment in patients suffering from pressure ulcers is not easy, because such ulcers are often found in elderly patients, who are frequently affected by multiple disorders and cognitive impairment (Dolynchuk *et al*, 2000). The evaluation of wound pain has, until now, been mainly based on reports coming from people living close to the patient. Visual analogue scales and numerical rating scales represent the two main tools in pain assessment. Deep infection is a frequent complication of grade III and grade IV pressure ulcers, and is characterised by an increase in warmth, tenderness, and pain (Sanada *et al*, 2006).

Dressing selection, application and removal

The selection of the dressing must be made in relation to the wound status and the surrounding skin condition. The aetiology of the wound also influences the dressing choice: for instance, a venous leg ulcer requires the use of a compression system over the dressing which may need to last up to seven days; a diabetic foot ulcer should be covered not only by the dressing, but, if neuropathic, also by an offloading system; a pressure ulcer should be treated with a pressure redistribution mattress or cushion. Moist wound healing is essential to avoid dry gauze from adhering to the wound bed, causing extreme discomfort while the dressing is on site and during the dressing change procedure. The frequency of dressing changes should be based on the caregiver's experience, in keeping with dressing characteristics and individual wound status. A less frequent dressing change could avoid potential trauma and pain for the patient. The caregiver must consider several aspects in making a decision at the time of dressing selection. He/she should consider the level of bacterial balance, match the amount of exudate with a proper dressing choice, recognise any potential allergy to products on the market, and be aware that the wound bed will change during treatment and that the dressing choice should follow, if possible, the progression of the tissue repair process. The depth of the wound is another important factor affecting dressing choice and prevention of wound pain. Full contact of the dressing with the wound bed should reduce the level of pain and protect the area from external agents.

The dressing should be applied following the manufacturer's instructions and should take into account the use of a secondary dressing (if required), and the role of extra fixation to hold the dressing in place for the necessary time. During this procedure, the surrounding skin could be protected with various products to avoid additional discomfort during treatment and at dressing removal.

Dressing removal is probably the most important procedure in relation to trauma and pain for the patient (Hollinworth and Collier, 2000). At this point, pain assessment should consider a brief history of the pain experienced by the patient during the previous two days, and any pain triggers during this intervention should be avoided. The positioning of the patient during dressing change is another aspect which may influence the outcome of the process. In an intensive care unit, with multiple devices working on a single patient, the dressing change-related procedure should follow a standardised protocol and every unnecessary manipulation of the wound should be avoided. The caregiver should reconsider the dressing choice if soaking is required for removal, or if removal is causing bleeding or trauma to the wound bed or to the surrounding skin. Several wound cleansers are currently available, but each product affects the level of pain differently, with potentially detrimental effects on wound healing. The method of delivering wound cleansers is also relevant for pain assessment and management, because such fluid can be used as a method of debridement in conjunction with other devices, or may be applied in a different way to preserve the new granulation tissue and epithelium.

Conclusion

Pain is a critical issue in wound management and strongly influences a patient's quality of life. Assessment of wound pain at dressing change is a fundamental part of wound care and must be accomplished in keeping with the patient's expectations. It is vital that practitioners are able to assess and manage pain using the principles of best practice currently available from various consensus documents. Pain assessment is an on-going procedure, which should involve a comprehensive investigation before, during and after every wound dressing-related action. Optimum local wound care influences pain assessment and the selection of an ideal wound dressing according to the status of the wound, and contributes to achieving positive outcomes and producing a faster healing response.

References

Caputo GM, Joshi N, Weitekamp MR (1997) Foot infections in patients with diabetes. *Am Fam Physician* **56**(1): 195–202

Dolynchuk K, Keast DH, Campbell KC *et al* (2000) Prevention and treatment of pressure ulcers. *Ostomy/Wound Management* **46**(11): 38–52

Eaglstein WH (1993) Occlusive dressings. *J Dermatol Surg Oncol* **19**(8): 716–20

European Wound Management Association (EWMA) (2002) *Position Document: Pain at wound dressing changes*. Medical Education Partnership Ltd, London

Frykberg RG (2002) Diabetic foot ulcers: pathogenesis and management. *Am Fam Physician* **66**(9): 1655–62

Hofman D, Ryan TJ, Arnold F *et al* (1997) Pain in venous leg ulcers. *J Wound Care* **6**(5): 222–4

Hollinworth H, Collier M (2000) Nurses views about pain and trauma at dressing changes: result of a national survey. *J Wound Care* **9**: 369–73

Lavery LA, Armstrong DG, Vela SA *et al* (1998) Practical criteria for screening patients at high risk for diabetic foot ulceration. *Arch Intern Med* **158**(2): 157–62

Meaume S, Teot L, Lazareth I *et al* (2004) The importance of pain reduction through dressing selection in routine wound management: the MAPP study. *J Wound Care* **10**(13): 409–13

Reddy M, Kohr R, Queen D *et al* (2003) Practical treatment of wound pain and trauma: a patient-centered approach. An overview. *Ostomy/Wound Management* **49**(4A): Suppl 2–15

Sanada H, Nakagami G, Romanelli M (2006) Identifying criteria for pressure ulcer infection. In: European Wound Management Association (EWMA) *Position Document: Identifying criteria for wound infection*. MEP Ltd, London

Schultz G, Mozingo D, Romanelli M *et al* (2005) Wound healing and TIME: new concepts and scientific applications. *Wound Rep Regen* **13**(4): S1–S13

Sibbald RG (1998) Venous leg ulcers. *Ostomy/Wound Management* **44**(9): 52–64

Winter GD (1962) Formation of the scab and the rate of epithelialization of superficial wounds in the skin of the young domestic pig. *Nature* **193**: 293–4

World Union of Wound Healing Societies (2004) *Principles of Best Practice: Minimising pain at wound dressing-related procedures. A consensus document.* Available online at: www.wuwhs.org/pdf/consensus_eng.pdf

CHAPTER 6

ALLERGIC REACTIONS TO TREATMENT

Janice Cameron

The management of chronic wounds involves the use of a range of topical treatments applied at different stages of the healing process. It is possible for a patient to become allergic to any part of their topical treatment, including dressings, emollients, creams and bandages, (Wilson *et al*, 1991). The number of allergic reactions seen in any one clinic or geographical area will often reflect local prescribing practices, product availability, or treatment preferences. An allergic response may influence the healing outcome by leading to breakdown of the surrounding skin and increased serous fluid loss. This can be distressing for the patient who may complain of burning, stinging and itching of the affected area, resulting from increased sensory stimulus to the skin. If an allergic reaction is suspected, an essential component of clinical decision-making in future patient management is identification of the causal agent (allergen). Changing the treatment alone is not enough, as this could re-expose the patient to the same allergen, which may be present in several different topical preparations (Cameron and Powell, 1992). In some patients, identification and subsequent allergen avoidance may result in the eczema resolving permanently.

Contact dermatitis

The terms eczema and dermatitis are now used synonymously. Eczema is an inflammatory reaction in the skin due to different causes. **Endogenous eczema** is the type of eczema that is related to constitutional factors such as atopic eczema. **Exogenous eczema** describes the type of eczema that is related to contact with external substances. Allergic contact dermatitis (ACD) and irritant contact dermatitis fall into this second group. Itchy skin is often a predominant symptom of both irritant and allergic contact dermatitis. If the patient then scratches the eczematous area, there is a risk of further loss of epithelium causing increased discomfort to the patient and delaying healing (Cameron, 1995a).

Allergic contact dermatitis (contact sensitivity)

The term 'dermatitis' comes from the Greek word *derma* (skin) and *itis* (inflammation). Allergic contact dermatitis, also known as contact sensitivity, is a delayed, type IV, hypersensitivity response activated by T-lymphocytes (Sibbald and Cameron, 2001). When an allergen comes into contact with the skin, allergen-bearing Langerhans cells from the skin, travel via the lymphatics to the draining lymph nodes, where they present the allergen to T-lymphocytes of the immune system. Specific T-cells proliferate to establish immunological memory. The memory T-cells mediate allergic contact dermatitis (Friedman, 1998). The activated (sensitised) lymphocytes produce mediators (eg. lymphokines), which enter the peripheral tissues and skin. On renewed contact with the allergen, these lymphocytes are reactivated via the skin and circulation, where they produce a response. This is seen clinically as inflamed skin, characterised by erythema, weeping, scaling and itching (allergic contact dermatitis) (Scheper and von Blomberg, 1992). This reaction is usually seen in the area of direct contact with the responsible allergen.

Contact sensitivity to topical applications is particularly common in patients who have chronic venous leg ulcers, with between 63% and 81% demonstrating a contact sensitivity relevant to the current or past ulcer treatment (Cameron, 1990; Wilson *et al*, 1991; Zaki *et al*, 1994; Gooptu and Powell, 1999; Marasovic and Vuksic, 1999; Tavadia *et al*, 2003; Machet *et al*, 2004; Saap *et al*, 2004). Many patients have multiple sensitivities, complicating local therapy considerably.

Venous leg ulcers often present with surrounding cutaneous changes, which may be the result of maceration or varicose eczema impairing the skin's natural barrier function. It is thought that the occlusive nature of dressings and bandages, on skin where the barrier function has been disturbed in this way, might create the perfect environment for developing contact sensitivity (Wilson *et al*, 1991). Some authors have found an association between the duration of the ulcer and the number of sensitivities, suggesting that patients with long-standing leg ulcers have a higher prevalence of sensitivity (Marasovic and Vuksic, 1999). It is possible that this may be purely due to increased exposure to potential sensitisers (Gallenkemper *et al*, 1998). If a contact allergy is suspected, the patient should be referred to a dermatologist for investigations as to the cause.

Investigations and diagnosis

Patch testing is an established method of investigating contact dermatitis with standardised methods for application and defined guidelines for reading and interpreting the results, recommended by the International Contact Dermatitis Research Group (ICDRG) (Wilkinson *et al*, 1970).

Various test systems are available commercially. Some tests come pre-prepared and ready to use. One commonly used system consists of strips of hypoallergenic tape (Scanpor tape), with small aluminium discs attached (Finn chambers). These are filled with small amounts of prepared allergens in a petroleum vehicle for testing. The original adhesive tape used for the patch tests was problematic, causing reactions in some patients. Subsequently, acrylate-based adhesive tapes were introduced and the problem has been virtually eliminated (Wahlberg, 1992).

Patch testing procedure

Most dermatologists would test to a standard series, topical series and corticosteroids, as well as patches reflecting local prescribing practices. The test strips are applied to healthy skin on the patient's upper back. After two days, the test strips are removed and the back examined. A further examination is undertaken two days later. These time points have been recommended as optimum for reading patch tests

(Paramsothy *et al*, 1988; Rietschel *et al*, 1988). At each examination, the degree of erythema, oedema, induration, and vesicle formation is recorded, and responses graded according to guidelines set down by the ICDRG.

Main leg ulcer allergens

Rubber accelerators — thiuram mix, carba mix

There appears to be a steady increase in sensitivity to rubber chemicals (Gooptu and Powell, 1999). Possible sources of rubber exposure include some elastic bandages and compression stockings. However, changes in nursing practice over the years have resulted in increasing use of rubber latex gloves, which may be associated with the apparent increase in sensitivity. Wearing vinyl gloves instead of rubber latex to treat leg ulcer patients may reverse this trend.

Topical antibiotics — neomycin, framycetin, gentamicin, bacitracin

Although neomycin and bacitracin are not related chemically, patients often become sensitised to both antibiotics simultaneously (Binnick and Clendinning, 1978; Zaki *et al*, 1994). Neomycin is a broad spectrum antibiotic of the aminoglycoside family. Cross-sensitivity occurs between neomycin, framycetin and gentamicin, and a positive reaction to one of the group means that they should all be avoided (Rudzki *et al*, 1988). A sensitivity reaction to neomycin may be masked in products where the antibiotic is combined with a corticosteroid, the latter suppressing the sensitivity reaction. A high number of sensitivities to gentamicin reported in one study were thought to reflect its increased use locally (Marasovic and Vuksic, 1999). Similarly, a high number of positive patch tests reported to bacitracin were also found to correspond to local prescribing habits (Zaki *et al*, 1994; Saap *et al*, 2004).

Fragrances — balsam of Peru/fragrance mix

Balsam of Peru is a natural substance obtained from fir trees. Balsam of Peru and fragrance mix are both markers of fragrance allergy, and can be found in creams, barrier preparations and bath additives. Both balsam of Peru and fragrance mix continue to be main sensitisers in leg ulcer patients (Marasovic and Vuksic, 1999; Reichert-Penetrat *et al*, 1999; Tavadia *et al*, 2003; Machet *et al*, 2004).

Lanolin — wool alcohols, Amerchol L 101

Lanolin is tested as wool alcohols and Amerchol L 101. Wool alcohols are the alcohol fraction of wool wax, a natural product from sheep fleece. They are emulsifying agents and emulsion stabilisers used in the preparation of creams and ointments. Although lanolin is not a potent sensitiser on normal skin, it remains a significant sensitiser in patients with varicose eczema and leg ulcers (Renna and Wollina, 2002; Machet *et al*, 2004). Lanolin is present in some barrier preparations, creams, bath additives and emollients used in the management of leg ulcers. It is also present in some over-the-counter products, including baby products, which may be used by the patients themselves. Lanolin is often listed in the product ingredient labelling as wool alcohols, and healthcare teams and patients may not always recognise this as being lanolin. Products containing lanolin, including newer lanolins which may also have a potential to sensitise, are best avoided around leg ulcers.

Emulsifiers — cetylstearyl alcohol (cetyl and stearyl alcohol)

Cetylstearyl alcohol is used in creams, ointments and other topical preparations as a stiffening agent and emulsion stabiliser. It is found in emollients such as aqueous cream and emulsifying ointment, and in most creams, including those used as direct ulcer applications. It is also present in some paste bandages and in corticosteroid creams (Cameron and Powell, 1992).

Adhesives — colophony/ester of rosin

Colophony is a widespread, naturally occurring material, which is obtained from tree rosin. Colophony and its derivatives can be found in the adhesive backing of some tapes, plasters, bandages and dressings. There have been a few reports of allergic reactions to hydrocolloid dressings. The patients involved also displayed positive patch tests to colophony (Mallon and Powell, 1994; Sasseville *et al*, 1997; Korber *et al*, 2006). However, failure to identify the responsible constituent in one hydrocolloid dressing has also been reported (Grange-Prunier *et al*, 2002).

Preservatives — parabens (hydroxybenzoates)

The parabens group of preservatives are widely used in topical preparations and possess antibacterial and antifungal properties.

Hydrogels

Sensitisation to hydrogels is becoming increasingly reported (Gallenkemper *et al*, 1998; Dawe *et al*, 2000; Tavadia *et al*, 2003; Lee and Kim, 2004). This is thought to be due to the ingredient propylene glycol, which is found in some hydrogels. Recent reports suggest propylene glycol is increasing in significance as a leg ulcer allergen (Saap *et al*, 2004).

Topical corticosteroids

As well as the excipients, the corticosteroid molecule itself may sensitise (Dunkel *et al*, 1991; Reichert-Penetrat *et al*, 1999; Tavadia *et al*, 2003; Gonul and Gul, 2005). Detection of the sensitivity can be difficult, as the anti-inflammatory effect of the corticosteroid may mask the contact allergy. Patients who are exhibiting a poor response to treatment with topical corticosteroids should be considered for patch testing.

Management of allergic contact dermatitis

Treatment is directed at controlling any eczema present and identifying the causal agent. Once an allergy has been identified, it is essential that the healthcare team and the patient themselves are aware of the allergy and its potential sources. Topical corticosteroids are the mainstay of treatment for eczema and are available as lotions, creams and ointments. Lotions may be applied to eczematous skin reactions under ostomy appliances. Creams are generally more suited to wet areas, and ointments to dry areas. Creams should be avoided on patients with chronic venous leg ulcers as they contain potential sensitisers, and ointments in a paraffin base should be used instead. The potency of the topical corticosteroid will depend on the severity of the eczema. Very potent and potent steroids should be used during the acute inflammatory stage of the reaction only, and reduced to a less potent preparation as soon as possible.

Irritant contact dermatitis

In some cases, the eczematous reaction may be an irritant response. Irritants may affect the skin in different ways, varying from slight scaling and erythema, to severe reactions with oedema, inflammation and vesiculation (Lisby and Baagsgaard, 2001). Dressings, bandages and even stockings can sometimes cause irritation and eczema. Without the benefit of patch testing, it is difficult to determine whether the skin reaction is an allergic or irritant contact dermatitis, as the clinical appearance is often indistinguishable. Irritant contact dermatitis was originally thought to be non-immunological, but recent findings have implicated the immune system in the development of irritant-induced contact dermatitis (Lisby and Baagsgaard, 2001). Irritants directly damage the keratin, impairing the barrier function of the skin. Patients often feel burning and stinging on direct contact with the irritant, compared with the delayed response of allergic contact dermatitis. Substances that may cause an irritant contact dermatitis used in wound management, or used by the patient themselves, include; antiseptics, adhesive tapes, adhesive dressings, some medicaments, moisturisers, soap and detergents.

Antiseptics

Many over-the-counter antiseptics have been shown to cause irritant skin reactions when applied to scratches on the forearms of volunteers (Patti _et al_, 1990).

Povidone-iodine preparations have been shown to be mainly irritant, but may also occasionally elicit an allergic response (Nishioka _et al_, 2000; Lachapelle, 2005). In the author's experience, application of povidone-iodine preparations to an open area can cause an immediate, sharp stinging in some patients.

Wound exudate

Wound exudate is a potential irritant. Chronic wound exudate contains raised levels of proteolytic enzymes that can damage healthy tissue (Trengove _et al_, 1999). Excessive exposure to wound exudate on previously healthy skin can result in enzymatic damage, leading to a reduction in the natural barrier function of the skin. Once the skin barrier function has been damaged, the patient is at risk from developing allergic contact dermatitis. The use of a suitable skin protectant applied to the peri-wound skin can prevent skin damage from wound exudate, and reduce the risk of further loss of epithelium (Cameron _et al_, 2005).

Dressings and bandages

Adhesive-backed tapes and dressings have been shown to remove varying amounts of superficial stratum corneum on removal from the skin. Some adhesive dressings have been found to elicit changes in the barrier function and superficial hydration of the skin (Zillmer _et al_, 2006). Continual, repeated application and removal may lead to an inflammatory skin reaction in some individuals (Dykes _et al_, 2001). The resulting clinical appearance of erythema, oedema and vesicular changes is similar to that of an allergic response. If this occurs, the skin will feel sore and there will be irritation. A further potential complication of adhesive-backed tapes and dressings is blistering.

This occurs when the epidermis becomes separated from the dermis due to excessive shear forces at the epidermis/dermis interface (Cosker *et al*, 2005). A barrier preparation that leaves a protective film on the skin surface may be applied under adhesive dressings to aid adhesion and prevent trauma on removal. Adhesive dressings are best avoided on eczematous skin and oedematous or fragile tissue.

Inappropriate use of dressings and bandages on a patient with weeping eczema may result in adhesion to the peri-wound skin, causing pain and trauma to the patient on removal. The patient then associates those particular dressings and bandages with pain and discomfort, and can sometimes confuse this with being allergic to the treatment.

Hosiery

Compression hosiery applied to patient's legs following healing may sometimes lead to skin irritation (Franks *et al*, 1993). This may cause patients to become reluctant to wear their stockings and increase the risk of ulcer recurrence. Simple interventions, like applying an emollient to prevent skin dryness, and applying a tubular cotton layer under the compression stocking, can help to reduce skin irritation (Cameron, 1995b).

Avoidance of allergens

Patients with eczema and other cutaneous changes, such as maceration, that impair the barrier function of the skin are at risk from developing an allergic reaction to their topical treatments. Identification of the responsible agent by patch testing and subsequent avoidance is an essential part of management that can limit unnecessary discomfort to the patient. Following patch testing, documentation of all positive patch test results should be readily available to both the patients and their carers. This should also include guidelines on how to avoid identified sensitisers in clinical practice. Leg ulcer allergens and their potential sources have been summarised in *Table 6.1*.

Before changes to the patient's wound and skin care treatment are instigated, any documentation regarding allergies should be consulted and relevant sensitivities noted. The ingredient labelling on the packaging can then be checked to identify if the relevant allergen is present before the treatment is applied to the patient. Where there is doubt as to the suitability of the product on a patient with known sensitivities, the company should be contacted for advice. Identification and subsequent avoidance of any responsible allergens will reduce the complications associated with an allergic contact dermatitis. The effect on the patient is an improvement in the condition and comfort of their skin, and sometimes, healing of the wound.

Table 6.1: Frequently reported allergens and their sources		
Type	Allergen used in testing to identify sensitivity	Potential sources
Rubber	Mercapto/carba/ thiuram mix	Elastic bandages, elastic stockings, latex gloves worn by carer
Perfume	Balsam of Peru/ fragrance mix	Bath oils, over-the-counter preparations, such as moisturisers and baby products
Topical antibiotics	Neomycin, framycetin, bacitracin, gentamicin	Antibiotic creams, ointments and dressings
Preservatives	Parabens (hydroxybenzoates)	Medicaments, creams and paste bandages
Adhesives	Colophony/ester of rosin	Adhesive-backed bandages and dressings
Lanolin	Wool alcohols, Amerchol L 101	Bath additives, creams, emollients, skin barriers and some baby products
Emulsifiers	Cetylstearyl alcohol	Most creams, including corticosteroid creams, direct ulcer applications, aqueous creams. Also present in emulsifying ointments and some paste bandages
Topical corticosteroids	Tixocortol pivalate	Steroid creams and ointments

Adapted from Cameron, 1995b

References

Binnick AN, Clendinning WE (1978) Bacitracin contact dermatitis. *Contact Dermatitis* 4: 180

Cameron J (1990) Patch testing for leg ulcer patients. *Nurs Times* 86(25): 63–4

Cameron J, Powell S (1992) Contact dermatitis: its importance in leg ulcer patients. *Wound Management* 2(3): 12–13

Cameron J (1995a) Contact sensitivity and eczema in leg ulcer patients. In: Cullum N, Roe B, eds. *Leg ulcers: Nursing management*. Scutari Press, London: 101–12

Cameron J (1995b) The importance of contact dermatitis in the management of leg ulcers. *J Tissue Viability* 5(2): 52–5

Cameron J, Hofman D, Wilson J, Cherry G (2005) Comparison of two peri-wound skin protectants in venous leg ulcers; a randomised controlled trial. *J Wound Care* 14(5): 233–6

Cosker T, Elsayed S, Gupta S *et al* (2005) Choice of dressing has a major impact on blistering and healing outcomes in orthopaedic patients. *J Wound Care* 14(1): 27–30

Dawe RS, Bianchi J, Douglas MB (2000) Allergic reactions to hydrogels. *J Wound Care* 8(4): 179 (letters)

Dunkel FG, Elsner P, Burg G (1991) Contact allergies to topical corticosteroids: 10 cases of contact dermatitis. *Contact Dermatitis* 25: 97–103

Dykes P, Heggie R, Hill SA (2001) Effects of adhesive dressings on the stratum corneum. *J Wound Care* 10(2): 7–10

Franks PJ, Oldroyd MI, Sharp EJ *et al* (1993) Factors associated with leg ulcer recurrence. In: Proceedings of the 3rd European Conference on Advances in Wound Management, Harrogate. Macmillan, London: 67

Friedman PS (1998) Allergy and the skin. II-Contact and atopic eczema. In: Durham SR, ed. *ABC of Allergies*. BMJ Books, London: 40–3

Gallenkemper G, Rabe E, Bauer R (1998) Contact sensitisation in chronic venous insufficiency: modern wound dressings. *Contact Dermatitis* 38: 274–8

Gonul M, Gul U (2005) Detection of contact hypersensitivity to corticosteroids in allergic contact dermatitis patients who do not respond to topical corticosteroids. *Contact Dermatitis* 53: 67–70

Gooptu C, Powell SM (1999) The problems of rubber hypersensitivity (Types I and IV) in chronic leg and stasis eczema patients. *Contact Dermatitis* 41: 89–93

Grange-Prunier A, Couilliet D, Grange F, Guillaume JC (2002) Allergic contact dermatitis to the Comfeel hydrocolloid dressing. *Ann Dermatol Venereol* **129**(5 Pt 1): 725–7 (original article in French)

Korber A, Kohaus S, Geisheimer M, Grabbe S, Dissemond J (2006) Allergic contact dermatitis from a hydrocolloid dressing due to colophony sensitization. *Hautarzt* **57**(3): 242–5 (original article in German)

Lachapelle JM (2005) Allergic contact dermatitis from povidone-iodine: a re-evaluation study. *Contact Dermatitis* **52**: 9–10

Lee JE, Kim SC (2004) Allergic contact dermatitis from a hydrogel dressing (Intrasite gel) in a patient with scleroderma. *Contact Dermatitis* **50**: 376–7

Lisby S, Baagsgaard O (2001) Mechanisms of irritant contact dermatitis. In: Rycroft RJG, Menné T, Frosch PJ, Lepoitteven JP, eds. *Textbook of Contact Dermatitis*. 3rd edn. Springer, Verlag. Berlin

Machet L, Couhe C, Perrinaud A *et al* (2004) A high prevalence of sensitisation still persists in leg ulcer patients: a retrospective series of 106 patients tested between 2001 and 2002 and a meta-analysis of 1975–2003 data. *Br J Dermatol* **150**(5): 929–35

Mallon E, Powell S (1994) Allergic contact dermatitis from Granuflex hydrocolloid dressing. *Contact Dermatitis* **30**: 110–11

Marasovic D, Vuksic I (1999) Allergic contact dermatitis in patients with leg ulcers. *Contact Dermatitis* **41**: 107–9

Nishioka K, Seguchi T, Yasuno H *et al* (2000) The results of ingredient patch testing in contact dermatitis elicited by povidone-iodine preparations. *Contact Dermatitis* **42**: 90–4

Paramsothy Y, Collins M, Smith AG (1988) Contact dermatitis in patients with leg ulcers. The prevalence of late positive reactions and evidence against systemic ampliative allergy. *Contact Dermatitis* **18**: 30–6

Patti J, Cazzaniga A, Marshall DA, Leyden JS, Mertz PM (1990) An analysis of dermal irritation of several OTC first aid treatments. *Wounds* **2**: 35–42

Reichert-Penetrat S, Barbaud A, Weber M, Schmutz JL (1999) Leg ulcers. Allergologic studies of 359 cases. *Ann Dermatol Venereol* **126**(2): 131–5

Renna R, Wollina U (2002) Contact sensitization in patients with leg ulcers and/or leg eczema: comparison between centers. *Lower Extremity Wounds* **1**(4): 251–5

Rietschel R, Adams RN, Mailbach HI (1988) The case for patch test readings beyond day 2. *J Am Acad Dermatol* **18**: 42–5

Rudzki E, Zakrzewski Z, Rebadel P *et al* (1988) Cross-reactions between aminoglycoside antibiotics. *Contact Dermatitis* **18**: 314–6

Saap L, Fahim S, Arsenault E *et al* (2004) Contact sensitivity in patients with leg ulcerations: a North American study. *Arch Dermatol* **140**(10): 1241–6

Sasseville D, Tennstedt D, Lapachelle JM (1997) Allergic contact dermatitis from hydrocolloid dressings. *Am J Contact Dermatitis* 8: 236–8

Scheper RJ, von Blomberg M (1992) Cellular mechanisms in allergic contact dermatitis. In: Rycroft RGJ, Menné T, Frosch PJ, Benezra C, eds. *Textbook of Contact Dermatitis*. Springer-Verlag, Berlin.

Sibbald RG, Cameron J (2001) Dermatological aspects of wound care. In: Krasner DL, Rodeheaver GT, Sibbald RG, eds. *Chronic Wound Care: A clinical source book for healthcare professionals*. 3rd edn. Wayne, PA: Health Management Publications Inc: 273–85

Tavadia S, Bianchi J, Dawe RS *et al* (2003) Allergic contact dermatitis in venous leg ulcer patients. *Contact Dermatitis* 48: 261–5

Trengove NJ, Stacey MC, MacAuley S *et al* (1999) Analysis of the acute and chronic wound environments: the role of proteases and their inhibitors. *Wound Rep Regen* 7: 42–52

Wahlberg JE (1992) Patch testing. In: Rycroft RGJ, Menné T, Frosch PJ, Benezra C, eds. *Textbook of Contact Dermatitis*. Springer-Verlag, Berlin

Wilkinson DS, Fregert S, Magnusson B *et al* (1970) Terminology of contact dermatitis. *Acta Dermatovener* (Stockholm) 50: 287–92

Wilson CL, Cameron J, Powell SM *et al* (1991) High incidence of contact dermatitis in leg ulcer patients — implications for management. *Clin Exp Dermatol* 16: 250–3

Zaki I, Shall L, Dalziel KL (1994) Bacitracin: a significant sensitiser in leg ulcer patients? *Contact Dermatitis* 31: 92–4

Zillmer R, Agren MS, Gottrup F, Karlsmark T (2006) Biophysical effects of repetitive removal of adhesive dressings on peri-ulcer skin. *J Wound Care* 15(5): 187–91

Table 6.2: Moisturisers, potential skin sensitisers as ingredients

	Fragrances	Beeswax	Cetyl/Cetostearyl/Stearyl alcohol	Propylene glycol	Triethanolamine	Lanolin/derivatives	Benzalkonium chloride	Benzyl alcohol	Hydroxybenzoates (parabens)	Phenethyl alcohol	Phenoxyethanol	Quarternium-15	Sorbic acid/sorbates	Triclosan	Butylated hydroxyanisole	Butylated hydroxytoluene	Other potential sensitisers
Alpha keri	•					•											❶
Aquadrate																	
Aveeno bath additive																	
Aveeno bath oil	•	•												•			
Aveeno cream			•					•									
Balneum bath oil	•			•												•	
Balneum plus cream								•									
Balneum plus oil	•		•													•	
Calmurid																	
Cetraben emollient bath additive																	
Cetraben emollient cream			•						•		•						
Dermalo bath emollient						•											
Dermamist																	
Dermol 200 shower emollient			•				•				•						❷
Dermol 500 lotion			•				•				•						
Dermol 600 bath emollient							•							•			

Table 6.2: Cont.

	Fragrances	Beeswax	Cetyl/Cetostearyl/Stearyl alcohol	Propylene glycol	Triethanolamine	Lanolin/derivatives	Benzalkonium chloride	Benzyl alcohol	Hydroxybenzoates (parabens)	Phenethyl alcohol	Phenoxyethanol	Quarternium-15	Sorbic acid/sorbates	Triclosan	Butylated hydroxyanisole	Butylated hydroxytoluene	Other potential sensitisers
Dermol cream							●										❷
Diprobase cream			●														❸
Diprobase ointment																	
Diprobath																	
Doublebase					●						●						
E45 bath oil																	
E45 cream			●			●			●								
E45 lotion						●		●	●								
E45 wash cream																	
Emulsiderm							●						●				
Epaderm			●														
Eucerin						●		●									
Eumobase		●	●														
Eurax cream	●	●	●		●				●	●							❹
Eurax lotion	●		●	●							●		●				❹
Gamma-derm		●	●	●					●		●		●				
Hydromol cream			●						●		●						
Hydromol emollient																	
Hydromol ointment																	
Imuderm	●														●		

Table 6.2: Cont.

	Fragrances	Beeswax	Cetyl/Cetostearyl/Stearyl alcohol	Propylene glycol	Triethanolamine	Lanolin/derivatives	Benzalkonium chloride	Benzyl alcohol	Hydroxybenzoates (parabens)	Phenethyl alcohol	Phenoxyethanol	Quarternium-15	Sorbic acid/sorbates	Triclosan	Butylated hydroxyanisole	Butylated hydroxytoluene	Other potential sensitisers
Infaderm	•													•			
Kamillosan		•				•			•								❺
Keri	•			•	•	•			•			•					
Lipobase			•						•								
Morhulin						•											
Nutraplus				•					•								
Oilatum cream			•	•				•					•				
Oilatum emollient	•					•											
Oilatum emollient fragrant free						•											
Oilatum gel	•																
Oilatum junior cream			•					•					•				
Oilatum plus						•	•							•			
Sprilon			•			•											
Sudocrem	•	•		•		•		•								•	*
Ultrabase cream	•		•						•								**
Unguentum M			•	•									•				
Vasogen						•					•						
Xepin			•					•									
Zerobase			•														❸

* Benzyl benzoate, benzyl cinnamate, ** Disodium edetate, ❶ Oxybenzone, ❷ Chlorhexidine, ❸ Chlorocresol,
❹ Crotamiton, ❺ Camomile extract

Section III: Aspects of wound trauma and pain

CHAPTER 7

PAIN IN VENOUS LEG ULCERS AND ITS IMPACT ON QUALITY OF LIFE

Valerie Douglas

It can be argued that, traditionally, there has been a misconception that venous leg ulcers are not painful. However, over the past decade a growing body of evidence has refuted this view by demonstrating that a significant number of patients with venous leg ulcers report moderate to severe pain. Quality of life studies have consistently highlighted that pain is an overwhelming issue for patients living with a leg ulcer, which profoundly affects their lives (Charles, 1995; Walshe, 1995; Douglas, 2001). This chapter explores the impact of painful venous leg ulcers on patients' quality of life and makes recommendations for improving patient care.

When examining the wider literature surrounding chronic pain, it is widely recognised that pain has the potential to impact upon every aspect of the pain sufferer's quality of life (Walker and Sofaer, 1998). Although the field of chronic pain management has evolved during the past 20 years, there has been a lack of literature in relation to recognising and managing chronic painful leg ulcers (Rook, 1997). In recent years, there has been a movement to address some of the issues surrounding wound pain, and a position document on wound pain has been published (European Wound Management Association [EWMA], 2002). This document, which involved eleven countries, confirmed that practitioners considered leg ulceration as the most painful wound to manage within clinical practice (Moffatt *et al*, 2002). Despite such recognition, another study demonstrated that healthcare professionals remain complacent and dismiss the level of pain that patients experience from their wound (Hollinworth and Collier, 2000). Furthermore, recent qualitative and quantitative studies suggest that issues surrounding painful leg ulcers are either frequently misunderstood, or ignored, both by formal and informal carers (Hofman *et al*, 1997; Douglas, 2001; King, 2003; Hareendran *et al*, 2005; Douglas, 2006).

The quantitative studies confirm that 88% of patients with venous leg ulcers experienced pain, which was particularly exacerbated by dressing changes (Noonan and Burge, 1998). These findings are consistent with an earlier study which challenged the traditional concept that only arterial leg ulcers were painful (Hofman *et al*, 1997). This study demonstrated that 64% of patients with a venous leg ulcer reported severe pain, while 38% of patients experienced continuous pain. Since these two studies illustrated the fact that venous leg ulcers can be very painful, there has been an increasing awareness to manage venous leg ulcer pain more effectively (Briggs and Torra i Bou, 2002). Nevertheless, recent qualitative studies suggest that there is still a lot of work to be done (Douglas, 2001; Hareendran *et al*, 2005; Douglas, 2006).

It has been well-documented that pain is a complex, subjective and perceptual individual phenomenon (Briggs and Torra i Bou, 2002), which may be significantly shaped by the individual's age, gender and emotional, social and cultural factors (Walding, 1991). Chronic pain has been defined as being progressive and episodic in nature, which can exert a powerful influence on personality and emotions (Karoly, 1985). When considering such complexities, it is of little surprise to learn that factors affecting venous ulcer pain and patient characteristics still remain largely unknown. Studies have acknowledged that compression bandaging, dressings, and subsequent dressing changes and leg position can contribute to pain (Hofman *et al*, 1997; Douglas, 2001). However, conversely, some studies have reported that leg elevation and compression therapy relieves pain (Hofman *et al*, 1997; Noonan and Burge, 1998; Douglas, 2001; Charles, 2004). In an attempt to understand factors associated with venous leg ulcer pain, a recent study explored the prevalence of pain in pure venous and mixed aetiology leg ulcers (Nemeth *et al*, 2003). This study identified four factors that statistically differentiated individuals with pain from those who had not experienced pain, and concluded that individuals with osteoarthritis or a foot ulcer, or those attending a leg ulcer service for a shorter period, or who had a lower mental health score were significantly more likely to experience pain. This Canadian study was, however, a longitudinal study conducted over three seasons, involving nurses who had received specialist training, and may not be transferable to the UK.

According to McCaffery (1983), pain is whatever the experiencing person says it is, and exists whenever he says it does. Such a definition is apt when considering qualitative research studies, as patients and their carers each have their own stories and experiences to tell (Charles, 1995; Walshe, 1995; Douglas, 2001; Hareendran *et al*, 2005; Douglas, 2006). It is imperative that healthcare professionals do not underestimate this rich qualitative data, as only the patient genuinely understands the significance of each experience (Price, 1996).

Qualitative research has clearly highlighted that venous leg ulcer pain is an overwhelming feature affecting patient's quality of life, which not only has a profound physical effect but also imposes significant psychological and social limitations on the patient and their carer(s) (Walshe, 1995; Douglas, 2001; Hareendran *et al*, 2005; Douglas, 2006). Sadly, some of these studies reported that patients frequently cited pain as the norm of having a leg ulcer, or as part of the ageing process, relating it either to previous personal experiences or their family history:

> *My mother suffered with ulcers… so, what can I expect.*
>
> (Douglas, 2001)

However, a recent study has demonstrated that with good wound management and effective compression therapy, patients' quality of life and their bodily pain improves significantly (Charles, 2004).

Physical impact of pain

Patients have described their pain as ranging from being an irritation, itching sensation to an intense, excruciating pain, the worst imaginable (Douglas, 2001; Hareendran *et al*, 2005). Patients frequently displayed and utilised non-verbal signs to describe their pain:

> *It's a sort of a going on and on pain… [long pause], always comes back no matter what you try.*
>
> (Douglas, 2001)

Not all patients attributed their pain directly to their ulcers. Various treatments were often the cause:

> *These new dressings sting like hell... but the nurse says they are really good dressings [long pause],... but the pain is worse.*
>
> (Douglas, 2001)

Similar findings have been reported previously (Walshe, 1995) with increasing emphasis on the importance of patient comfort during treatments. There is now a wide range of wound dressings and treatment options available to practitioners, which was clearly recognised by some patients:

> *Nurses try this and that... every week a new dressing, nothing gets chance to work, the pain just persists.*
>
> (Douglas, 2001)

The past few years has seen a surge of dressings available on Drug Tariff. This was certainly evident within the qualitative studies and supports the view that there still appears to be much confusion about the properties of dressings (Hollinworth and Collier, 2000). The breadth of knowledge needed to inform clinical and professional practice within wound care is both complex and demanding (Flanagan, 2000). Hollinworth and Collier (2000) reinforce this view, stating that as nurses we have a duty to understand the properties of various dressing products, urging practitioners to use this as a key strategy in reducing patient pain at dressing changes:

> *I just kept telling the nurse it was too painful... but she insisted it was the right treatment as she had just done a study day on it... after she left I take it all off.*
>
> (Douglas, 2001)

Such misunderstandings and poor concordance will only lead to inappropriate pain control and weaken the patient–nurse relationship. Patients and carers frequently admitted that they felt that they could not report pain for fear of being labelled difficult or complaining (Douglas, 2001; Douglas, 2006). Despite the term compliance being replaced with the term concordance, practitioners continue to label non-concordant patients as 'deviant' or 'difficult' (Moffatt, 2004). In the past, practitioners have often viewed non-concordant behaviour as problematic, as it contravenes professional beliefs, norms and expectations (Playe and Keeley, 1998), which only leads to increased feelings of exasperation and frustration by both parties involved (Moore, 1995).

Furthermore, a study, which explored patient and professional dilemmas in non-healing, demonstrated that healthcare professionals continue to struggle with the realities of leg ulcer management, and often blame non-healing ulcers largely on issues of non-concordance (Moffatt, 2001).

Maintaining effective pain control can present difficulties for patients. The analgesia prescribed is often inadequate or not taken at all (Douglas, 2001; Hareendran *et al*, 2005; Hofman *et al*, 1997), with patients expressing that no one really understands their need for analgesia. Pain subsequently affects mobility, as standing and walking tend to aggravate the patient's leg ulcer pain (Walshe, 1995; Noonan and Burge, 1998; Douglas, 2001). Such immobility will inevitably have a direct impact on venous leg ulcer healing (Franks *et al*, 1995).

Pain was frequently cited as the causative factor for many sleepless nights (Douglas, 2001; Hareendran *et al*, 2005):

[It] keeps me awake all night... I toss and turn.

(Douglas, 2001)

Another study confirmed that 64% of patients with venous leg ulcers suffered sleep disturbance (Hofman *et al*, 1997). It has been well-documented that sleep deprivation impairs tissue formation, which can delay wound healing (North, 1990). However, a recent study highlighted that it is not just patients who have sleepless nights as a consequence of leg ulcer pain (Douglas, 2006), but that their carers felt 'continuously exhausted'. Many reported that they were unable to sleep, attributing this to 'being on call', knowing that they would be disturbed by their spouse's pain. Such sleep deprivation creates a negative state of well-being, and will have an inevitable psychological impact upon the patient and carer (Closs, 1992):

Sometimes we have bad nights from the ulcer... and I have
to get up.

(Douglas, 2006)

Psychological impact of pain

Qualitative studies have reported that unresolved leg ulcer pain leads to patients and their carers experiencing heightened anxieties, with feelings of irritability, frustration, and anger expressed (Krasner, 1998; Douglas, 2001; Hareendran *et al*, 2005; Douglas, 2006). Feelings of anxiety and depression, with associated negative feelings of self, have been well-documented within the chronic pain literature (Sternbach, 1978; Walker and Sofaer, 1998).

Patients and their carers living with chronic, painful leg ulcers have frequently expressed feelings of helplessness and loss of control (Charles, 1995; Douglas, 2001; Ebbeskog and Ekman, 2001; Douglas, 2006). Earlier work indicates that patients living with chronic pain portray the belief that no one is able to help them (Skevington, 1983), with another study reporting that patients with chronic pain dwell on regrets from their past which are unrelated to their pain, and experience personal relationship difficulties (Walker and Sofaer, 1998). Sternbach (1978) suggests that an individual's personality may influence their degree of pain and coping strategies. As pain is such a private experience, a range of coping strategies and methods of adapting have been demonstrated by patients and their carers (Krasner, 1998; Douglas, 2001; Douglas, 2006). Effective coping strategies require the patient to appraise their own circumstances and to utilise resources to meet their needs (Lazarus, 1985). One patient, who focused on work as a coping strategy, reported:

> *[I] kept working, working all the hours in the day… when I did stop, the pain was back with vengeance.*

(Douglas, 2001)

Krasner (1998) reminds us that being chronically ill with a painful venous leg ulcer is a different way of being in the world than being healthy — it is not just the patient's life that is affected. Informal carers have their own stories to share, relating their married life to like 'living with a leg ulcer' (Douglas, 2006):

> *Each day is like walking on eggshells… you just never know how things will be [biting her tongue].*

(Douglas, 2001)

*I just feel so angry all the time... so fed up with his pain and
depressed at the whole situation... intolerable at times... I can
cope caring with the physical bits, but the psychological bits... it's
just so soul destroying... [continuously wrenching his hands].*

(Douglas, 2006)

Although all the carers within this study were committed to caring
for their partners, they each expressed a sense of extreme worry and
concern about their partner's painful leg ulcers:

*I used to be quite a placid person... [long pause]... now life seems
to be one big worry about these ulcers.*

(Douglas, 2006)

*I just cry and cry at times... feel helpless... just could not stop...
so fed up with myself... just did not know which way to turn...
now on antidepressants.*

(Douglas, 2006)

The emotional burden of informal caring cannot be underestimated,
and has previously been reported as constantly emotionally draining
and intense (Highet *et al*, 2004). A study by Henwood (1998) reported
that 52% of carers had been treated with a stress-related disorder.
Carers looking after their spouses with a painful leg ulcer frequently
stated that they felt stressed and equated their experiences with
examples like 'living on the edge', or 'where has the light gone from
the tunnel?' (Douglas, 2006).

Social aspects of pain

Leg ulcer pain takes a central place in a patient's life, having a significant
impact on both the patient and carer's social life (Douglas, 2001; 2006;
Ebbeskog and Ekman, 2001). The patient's ulcer becomes the focal
point in their lives, not only restricting their daily activities, but also
resulting in the patient and their carer withdrawing from society.
According to Hareendran *et al* (2005), 97% of patients living with a
leg ulcer had some restriction to their every day functioning, with 38%
reporting that their social life was restricted by leg ulcer pain.

Leading such a restrictive life has led to patient's expressing feelings of isolation (Douglas, 2001), and carers feeling imprisoned or trapped within their own homes:

Life is just so restrictive now... live within these four walls, like a prisoner really.

(Douglas, 2006)

The theme of social isolation has been well-documented in the literature surrounding chronic illness and the elderly (Hodges *et al*, 2001). It is of little surprise to learn that patients and their informal, elderly carers felt so isolated. Informal carers expressed feelings of guilt and displayed signs of withdrawing from social events, or doing hobbies outside of the home (Douglas, 2006). Another study, which presented the theme 'a shrinking life', represented feelings of isolation and entrapment (Ohman and Soderberg, 2004). These findings are consistent with other studies, with carers in some instances staying at home and ceasing their hobbies to avoid conflict with their partner (Hutto Faria, 1998).

Unemployment, with associated feelings of 'loss of social role', has been reported within leg ulcer studies, with pain being the attributing factor (Phillips *et al*, 1994; Douglas, 2001). A quantitative study demonstrated a strong correlation between leg ulceration and job loss, with 42% of non-working patients claiming that their ulcer was the significant factor in stopping work (Phillips *et al*, 1994). Employment is heavily viewed as an important social role within society (Pugliesi, 1995). This study, which sampled 1352 people in employment, confirmed a positive association between social integration at work and self-esteem, and concluded that social integration increases happiness, particularly among the female workforce. The literature also suggests that women with chronic illness are more likely to suffer social isolation and financial hardship (McDonough *et al*, 1995). Such adjustments and increased dependency create feelings of helplessness, which leads to increased levels of psychological distress (Walker and Sofaer, 1998).

A recent study demonstrated that delivering care within a social setting as opposed to a conventional approach, statistically improved patients' leg ulcer pain, mood and sleep (Edwards *et al*, 2005). This study concluded that such findings have implications for healthcare professionals providing care for patients with leg ulcers. However, such an approach to leg ulcer services presents challenges for healthcare professionals within the ever-changing, turbulent, political climate of the NHS as, in many areas, primary care trusts are currently withdrawing leg ulcer clinics due to financial limitations.

This chapter has reviewed the literature surrounding leg ulcer pain and highlighted some of the physical, psychological and social implications. Uncontrolled leg ulcer pain leads to loss of independence, feelings of loss of control, low self-esteem and increased dependency.

Recommendations

In wound care, it is imperative that accurate pain assessment is undertaken by a competent healthcare professional, which incorporates a visual pain assessment tool and considers:

- when the pain is experienced
- the duration of the pain
- the type of pain, intensity
- any specific pain characteristics or co-morbidities to that patient.

Such a tool gives patients the opportunity to express their pain and provides practitioners with documented evidence of the efficacy or failure of any therapy implemented (Carr and Mann, 2000).

A pain diary is invaluable, as such recordings will provide a detailed account of the pattern of the patient's pain, highlight any attributing factors, and identify strategies to relieve pain (Hollinworth, 2005). By listening attentively to patients' pain experiences, practitioners will also be able to observe and record non-verbal signs of pain, which helps patients to feel valued as an individual (Hollinworth and Hawkins, 2002).

The management of pain is dependent on the diagnosis of the pain source (Ryan *et al*, 2003). When assessing leg ulcer pain, practitioners need to distinguish between nociceptive pain, which presents as a nagging, throbbing, gnawing type of pain, as opposed to neuropathic pain, which is often described as a shooting, burning, aching pain or the sensation of pins and needles (*Chapter 2*). Once the type of leg ulcer pain has been established, appropriate, effective and regular analgesia is recommended to meet these specific characteristics and patients' individual needs (*Chapter 8*).

It has not always been acknowledged that associated skin conditions, eg. irritant varicose eczema can give rise to pain (Douglas, 2001). To reduce pain, the dermatological aspects of leg ulceration should be addressed with the use of emollients and topical steroids where appropriate. Another factor in the patient's pain experience is oedema, which needs a multidisciplinary approach to resolve (Ryan *et al*, 2003).

An effective pain management approach is to empower patients to actively take control of their pain (Adams and Field, 2001). It has already been established within the literature that improved communication enhances a patient's sense of control, and that withdrawal, or lack of information, leads to perceived difficult behaviour (English and Morse, 1988). It is imperative that a collaborative and participatory relationship with patients and their carers is adopted, which will promote self-control, improve self-esteem, and encourage patients and their carers to develop active coping strategies (Douglas, 2001; Douglas, 2006).

Edwards *et al* (2005) proposed an alternative approach to conventional leg ulcer care, with the study demonstrating that such an approach empowers patients, enhances quality of life and reduces leg ulcer pain. With the proposed changes within the NHS, healthcare professionals could grasp this opportunity by developing a business plan to promote a social model of leg ulcer care.

Two position documents which offer practical advice for clinicians have been published on managing pain at dressing changes (EWMA, 2002; World Union of Wound Healing Societies [WUWHS], 2004). Furthermore, another review has urged that the current national leg ulcer guidelines be adjusted to reflect patient specific problems (Persoon *et al*, 2004). These papers recommend a multidisciplinary, collaborative approach to pain relief, which includes the involvement of a pain specialist nurse, when necessary. As accountable practitioners, we need to ensure that we keep up-to-date with such guidelines, and that clinical practice is standardised and evidence-based (McMullen, 2004).

Suggested strategies for reducing pain at dressing change include: (Briggs and Torra i Bou, 2002; Hollinworth, 2005):

* Involving and empowering the patient as much as possible.
* Pre-medicating prior to dressings if necessary.
* Encouraging slow rhythmic breathing during dressing changes.

❖ Encouraging patients to control the pace of the procedure, offer 'time out'.

❖ Reassuring the patient and adopting a calm, confident approach.

❖ Avoiding any unnecessary stimulus to the ulcer, such as prodding, poking on application of dressings and bandages; handling wounds and surrounding skin gently, especially if atrophie blanche is present as this can cause severe, sharp pain (Ryan *et al*, 2003).

❖ Using warm cleansing solutions before irrigating the wound.

❖ Ensuring correct application of dressings and bandages according to manufacturer's guidelines.

❖ Selecting atraumatic dressings which will:
  • minimise pain and trauma on removal
  • promote moist wound healing and reduce friction at the wound surface
  • remain *in situ* for longer periods to reduce the need for frequent dressing changes.

A review of the scientific and clinical literature surrounding soft silicone Safetac Technology confirmed that such products are atraumatic and can be used safely in all wound types (White, 2005). The wound care industry are becoming increasingly aware of the need to develop dressings to reduce pain, with a recent study confirming that hydrogel sheets reduce leg ulcer pain (Young and Hampton, 2005).

Non-pharmacological interventions, in conjunction with pharmacological treatments, can also be considered during dressing changes. Studies have demonstrated that diversional and relaxation therapies (Melzack and Wall, 1988), and distraction through interactive, computerised virtual reality (Hoffman *et al*, 2000) reduces wound pain.

To summarise, there is limited research surrounding effective management of painful venous leg ulcers (Heinen *et al*, 2004) and factors relating to venous pain still remain poorly understood. There is, therefore, an urgent need for further research within this field, and for the wound care industry to work in conjunction with practitioners to develop products which will reduce wound pain.

It is imperative that we, as practitioners, actively engage with our patients and listen to their pain experiences. If pain remains unresolved or is inflicted on patients as a result of dressing changes, this will create ethical and professional tensions (Hollinworth, 2005), which will inevitably have an impact on the nurse–patient relationship and affect concordance. Working in close collaboration will ultimately improve quality of life for both patients and carers.

References

Adams N, Field L (2001) Pain management 1: psychological and social aspects of pain. *Br J Nurs* **10**(14): 903–11

Briggs M, Torra i Bou JE (2002) *Pain at wound dressing changes: a guide to management.* European Wound Management Association Position Document: Pain at wound dressing changes. Medical Education Partnership, London.

Carr EC, Mann EM (2000) *Pain: Creative Approaches to Effective Management.* Macmillan Press Ltd, Basingstoke

Charles H (1995) The impact of leg ulcers on patients' quality of life. *Prof Nurse* **10**(9): 571–4

Charles H (2004) Does leg ulcer treatment improve patients' quality of life? *J Wound Care* **13**(6): 209–13

Closs SJ (1992) Patient's night time pain, analgesic provision and sleep after surgery. *Int J Nurs Stud* **29**(4): 381–92

Douglas V (2001) Living with a chronic leg ulcer: an insight into patients' experiences and feelings. *J Wound Care* **10**(9): 355–60

Douglas V (2006) *Living with a Leg Ulcer: From a carer's perspective.* Unpublished MSc Thesis. University of Hertfordshire

Ebbeskog B, Ekman SL (2001) Elderly persons' experiences of living with venous leg ulcer: living in a dialectal relationship between freedom and imprisonment. *Scand J Caring Sci* **15**: 235–43

Edwards H, Courtney M, Finlayson K, Lewis C, Lindsay E Shuter P, Chang A (2005) Chronic venous leg ulcers: effect of a community nursing intervention on pain and healing. *Nurs Standard* **19**(52): 47–54

English J, Morse J (1988) The 'difficult' elderly patient: adjustment or maladjustment? *J Nurs Stud* **25**(1): 23–9

European Wound Management Association (EWMA) (2002) *Position Document: Pain at wound dressing changes.* Medical Education Partnership Ltd, London

Flanagan M (2000) The responsibility is yours. *J Wound Care* **9**(8): 357

Franks PJ, Bosanquet N, Connolly M, Oldroyd M, Moffatt CJ, Greenhalgh RM, McCollum CN (1995) Venous ulcer healing: effect of socio-economic factors in London. *J Epidemiol Community Health* **49**(4): 385–8

Hareendran A, Bradbury A, Budd J, Geroulakos G, Hobbs R, Kenkre J, Symonds T (2005) Measuring the impact of venous leg ulcers on quality of life. *J Wound Care* **14**(2): 53–7

Heinen MM, van Achterberg T, Scholte op Reimer W, van de Kerkhof P, de Laat E (2004) Venous leg ulcer patients: a review of the literature on lifestyle and pain-related interventions. *J Clin Nurs* **13**: 355–66

Henwood M (1998) *Ignored and Invisible? Carers' Experience of the NHS.* Carers National Association, London

Highet NJ, McNair BG, Davenport TA, Hickie IB (2004) 'How much more can we lose?': carer and family perspectives on living with a person with depression. *Med J Aust* **181**(7): S6–S9

Hodges HF, Keeley AC, Grier EC (2001) Masterworks of art and chronic illness experiences in the elderly. *J Adv Nurs* **36**(3): 389–98

Hoffman HG, Patterson DR, Carrougher GJ (2000) Use of virtual reality for adjunctive treatment of adult burn pain during physical therapy: a controlled study. *Clin J Pain* **16**(3): 244–50

Hofman D, Ryan TJ, Arnold F, Cherry GW, Lindholm C, Bjellerup M, Glynn C (1997) Pain in venous leg ulcers. *J Wound Care* **6**(5): 222–4

Hollinworth H (2005) Pain at wound dressing-related procedures: a template for assessment. Available online at: www.worldwidewounds. com/2005/august/Hollinworth/Framework-Assessing-Pain (accessed 1 May 2006)

Hollinworth H, Collier M (2000) Nurses' views about pain and trauma at dressing changes: results of a national survey. *J Wound Care* **9**(8): 369–73

Hollinworth H, Hawkins J (2002) Teaching nurses psychological support of patients with wounds. *Br J Nurs* **11**(20): S8–S18

Hutto Faria S (1998) Through the eyes of a family caregiver: perceived problems. *Home Care Provider* **3**(4): 221–5

Karoly P (1985) The assessment of pain: concepts and procedures. In: Karoly P, ed. *Management Strategies in Health Psychology.* John Wiley, New York: 119–36

King B (2003) A review of research investigating pain and wound care. *J Wound Care* **12**(6): 219–23

Krasner D (1998) Painful venous ulcers: themes and stories about their impact on quality of life. *Ostomy/Wound Management* **44**(9): 38–49

Lazarus RS (1985) Coping theory and research: past, present and future. *Psychosom Med* **55**: 237–47

McCaffery M (1983) *Nursing the Patient in Pain.* Harper Row, London

McDonough PA, Badley EM, Tennant A (1995) Disability, resources, role demands and mobility handicap. *Disabil Rehabil* **17**: 159–68

McMullen M (2004) The relationship between pain and leg ulcers: a critical review. *Br J Nurs* **13**(19): S30–S36

Melzack R, Wall PD (1988) *The Challenge of Pain.* 2nd edn. Penguin Books, London

Moffatt CJ (2001) Patient and professional dilemmas in non-healing. Abstract presented at: Symposium on Advanced Wound Care and Medical Research Forum on Wound Repair. Las Vegas, Nevada, 30 April –3 May

Moffatt CJ, Franks PJ, Hollinworth H (2002) *Understanding wound pain and trauma: an international perspective*. European Wound Management Association Position Document: Pain at wound dressing changes. Medical Education Partnership Ltd, London

Moffatt CJ (2004) Perspectives on concordance in leg ulcer management. *J Wound Care* **13**(6): 243–8

Moore KN (1995) Compliance or collaboration? The meaning for the patient. *Nurs Ethics* **2**(1): 71–7

Nemeth KA, Harrison MB, Graham ID, Burke S (2003) Pain in pure and mixed aetiology venous leg ulcers: a three phase point prevalence study. *J Wound Care* **12**(9): 336–40

Noonan L, Burge SM (1998) Venous leg ulcers: is pain a problem? *Phlebology* **13**:14–19

North A (1990) The effect of sleep on wound healing. *Ostomy/Wound Management* March/April: 57–58

Ohman M, Soderberg S (2004) The experiences of close relatives living with a person with serious chronic illness. *Qual Health Res* **14**(3): 396–410

Persoon A, Heinen M, van der Vleuten C, Rooij M, van de Kerkhof P, van Achterberg (2004) Leg ulcers: a review of their impact on daily life. *J Clin Nurs* **13**: 341–54

Phillips T, Stanton B, Provan A, Lew R (1994) A study of the impact of leg ulcers on quality of life: Financial, social and psychologic implications. *J Am Acad Dermatol* **31**: 48–53

Playle JF, Keeley P (1998) Non-compliance and professional power. *J Adv Nurs* **27**(2): 304–11

Price P (1996) Quality of life meeting. *J Wound Care* **5**(3): 103

Pugliesi K (1995) Work and well-being: gender differences in the psychological consequences of employment. *J Health Soc Behav* **36**: 57–71

Rook JL (1997) Wound care pain management. *Nurse Practitioner* **22**(3): 122–36

Ryan S, Eager C, Sibbald RG (2003) Venous leg ulcer pain. *Ostomy/Wound Management* **49**(4A): 16–23

Skevington SM (1983) Chronic pain and depression: universal or personal helplessness. *Pain* **15**: 309–17

Sternbach RA (1978) Clinical aspects of pain. In: Sternbach RA, ed. *The Psychology of Pain*. Raven, New York: 62–70

Walding MF (1991) Pain, anxiety and powerlessness. *J Adv Nurs* **16**(4): 388–97

Walker J, Sofaer B (1998) Predictors of psychological distress in chronic pain patients. *J Adv Nurs* **27**(2): 320–6

Walshe C (1995) Living with a venous leg ulcer: a descriptive study of patients' experiences. *J Adv Nurs* **22**(6): 1092–1100

White R (2005) Evidence for atraumatic soft silicone wound dressing use. *Wounds UK* **1**(3): 104–9

World Union of Wound Healing Societies (2004) *Principles of Best Practice: Minimising pain at wound dressing-related procedures. A consensus document*. Available online at: www.wuwhs.org/pdf/consensus_eng.pdf

Young SR, Hampton S (2005) Pain management in leg ulcers using Actiform Cool®. *Wounds UK* **1**(3): 94–101

CHAPTER 8

MEDICAL MANAGEMENT OF CHRONIC WOUND PAIN

R Gary Sibbald, Adam Katchky and Douglas Queen

The study of pain in chronic wounds is in its infancy and there is a paucity of evidence to guide the clinician. Chronic wounds require complex care because they have a have a myriad of causes and complications.

The 'preparing the wound bed management paradigm' (previously developed by Sibbald *et al*, 2003b) is a basis for the management of chronic wounds and has been used extensively by wound care specialists. It consists of four major principles:

1. Treating the cause.
2. Addressing patient-centred concerns.
3. Providing local wound care.
4. Using advanced therapies when the wound is not healing at the expected rate.

We have integrated the management of chronic wound pain into this wound management paradigm (*Figure 8.1*). Treating the cause should involve determining the correct diagnosis and initiating appropriate wound pain treatment. Patient-centred concerns must focus on what the patient perceives as the disability caused by the pain, and their willingness to receive treatment. Local wound care needs to revolve around the three pillars of local wound care practice: debridement, bacterial balance/prolonged inflammation, and moisture balance.

The 'preparing the wound bed management paradigm' provides a foundation on which we have built a structured approach to optimise pain management in chronic wounds.

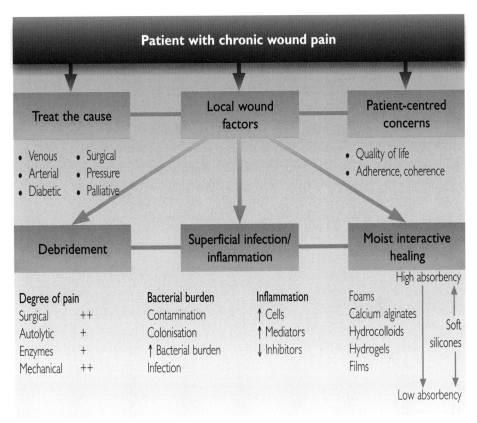

Figure 8.1: Chronic wound pain paradigm. Adapted from Sibbald *et al*, 2003, Reddy *et al*, 2003

General approach to chronic wound pain

Treat the cause

Treating the cause of a chronic wound may involve removing the source of the problem, for example with a venous ulcer, we are removing the oedema with compression therapy. This will be discussed further when the types of chronic wounds are discussed more specifically.

Patient-centred concerns

Pain in chronic wounds is a major concern for patients and healthcare professionals (Sibbald, 1998; Neil and Munjas, 2000). In a recent survey of 210 long-term care nurses and nurses who spend 50% of their time in wound care, pain was identified as the third biggest issue after time to healing and limb preservation (Eager, 2005). The patients in this same survey identified pain and quality of life issues as their first concern. Pain control is often more important to patients than it is to healthcare professionals (Queen *et al*, 2005).

Local wound care

Dressing removal is usually cited as the time when the most pain occurs. Dried out dressings and adherent products are most likely to cause pain and trauma at dressing changes, with gauze removal being the most common cause of this pain. Newer products, such as soft silicone dressings, hydrogels, Hydrofiber® (ConvaTec), and alginates are less likely to cause pain (Hollinworth and Collier, 2000).

Debridement

Wound debridement can be achieved through surgical, autolytic, enzymatic, and/or mechanical means (Davies *et al*, 2005). A number of factors come into play when choosing an appropriate debridement method. Each method can have a negative or positive impact on wound pain. The more aggressive the debridement regime (eg. surgical and mechanical), the more potential pain for the patient. In the presence of neuropathy, surgical debridement may be painless, unless deeper structures such as bone are disrupted. Enzymatic and autolytic debridements are slower but are generally less painful, with autolytic methods being essentially pain free.

For surgical debridement, application of topical local anaesthetics, such as 4% topical lidocaine, amethocaine 4% gel or EMLA, 30–60 minutes prior to the procedure may be helpful. For deeper debridement, injected local anaesthetics should be used. Even though spinal cord injured patients are often insensate in the debridement area, injected local anaesthetics should be used to avoid autonomic dysreflexia that can cause catastrophic elevations in blood pressure or muscle spasms (Weaver *et al*, 2006). If oral pain medications are used, the agents should be administered 30–90 minutes prior to debridement to obtain a therapeutic effect.

Non-pharmacological interventions are also important for debridement. These interventions include proper positioning prior to the procedure and creating a relaxed environment for the patient by making them comfortable and giving them a sense of control by allowing them to call a time-out. Pain intensity should be measured with a pain intensity scale, and the roles and responsibilities for pain management should be clarified prior to debridement (Davies *et al*, 2005). Environmental pain control strategies include guided imagery, talking to a supportive person, warm sheets, and the ability to call an agreed time-out when the pain reaches a predetermined level.

Superficial infection/inflammation

Infection and inflammation can be painful in themselves (Gardner *et al*, 2001). Superficial infections may be treated with topical antimicrobials, while deeper infections require systemic agents (Krasner and Sibbald, 1999). Many topical preparations, both pharmacological and non-pharmacological (eg. antibacterial dressings), exist to treat both infection and inflammation. Silver-containing dressings are both anti-inflammatory and antimicrobial (Wright *et al*, 2002). Acute inflammation is an important phase in normal healing and, therefore, treatment should be used only in cases of chronic inflammation (Bowler, 2002; 2003). Many of these preparations can be soothing or cooling (ointments/gels), or can create an appropriate environment to reduce or prevent pain (eg. moist dressings).

Deep infection

It has been shown in numerous studies that chronic wound exudate has an abnormally high concentrations of proteases (particularly matrix metalloproteinases, or MMPs) (Mast and Schultz, 1996). These increased proteases shift the wound healing balance into a continuing chronic inflammatory phase. Continued inflammation and tissue injury contributes to chronic wound pain and prevents the wound from transitioning to the proliferative stage. Increased pain in the area of an ulcer is a sign of possible deep infection. The mnemonic: STONES (Size increasing, Temperature elevated, O for probing to bone, New areas of breakdown, E for erythema, exudate edema and Smell) and ulcers that probe to bone should be investigated for osteomyelitis. Superficial bacterial burden can be identified with the mnemonic NERDS (Non-healing, Exudate, Red friable granulation, Debris on the surface or Smell). To identify bacterial damage, usually two or three of these symptoms need to be present. This can often be treated topically but if deep- or surrounding skin-invasion is present, the use of appropriate systemic antibiotics is required (Sibbald *et al*, 2003b). Exudate is often clear before it is frankly purulent. In the presence of exudate and odour, other signs of deep infection are used to clarify if bacterial damage involves the deep compartment as well. Treatment of bacterial invasion often leads to improvement in pain as the infection resolves.

Moist interactive healing

Moist wound healing has been demonstrated to result in faster healing, less scarring, and less pain (Rovee, 1991; Kannon and Garrett, 1995). The pain reduction has been attributed to the bathing of the exposed nerve ending in fluid, preventing dehydration of the nerve receptors.

Other dressing-related factors that can cause pain, include the dressing absorbency mechanism, dressing adherence, and the presence of contact irritants and allergens within the dressing (*Chapter 6*).

The manner in which a dressing absorbs and manages exudate can also result in wound pain. Dressing adherence to the wound can occur if the dressing absorbs too aggressively, or if the primary dressing allows secondary products to adhere to the wound. Adhesion of primary and secondary products can result in the accidental traumatic removal of the primary contact layer, resulting in damage to the wound bed and pain (World Union of Wound Healing Societies [WUWHS], 2004).

Fibrous products (eg. alginates, Hydrofiber®) are excellent primary contact layers. In the presence of wound fluid, these fibres transform into gels to facilitate a moist interactive local wound bed environment and result in a soothing sensation. The retained moisture facilitates non-traumatic removal and generally provides pain relief. Some dressings are abrasive and can cause local friction with movement or adherence to the wound surface (eg. some traditional gauze-based products). This can be avoided with the appropriate choice of primary dressings (eg. gels/foams), or the utilisation of an atraumatic wound contact layer (eg. soft silicone dressings) (Meuleneire, 2002).

Adhesive dressings, as the name suggests, can be traumatic to both the wound bed and peri-wound areas. Their removal can be both painful and damaging depending on the force necessary to remove the dressing. Films and hydrocolloids should be removed with care and as recommended by the manufacturer's instructions. To minimise adhesive trauma at dressing change, healthcare professionals are encouraged to stretch the dressing laterally, loosening the adhesive bond before exerting an upward vertical force away from the skin surface.

Hydrocolloids are generally non-adherent where the contents have gelled and interacted with the surface of the wound bed. They form a soft, conforming gel in the presence of exudate (Fletcher, 2005). However, upon removal, care should be taken to ensure that there is no skin stripping where the adhesive is fixed to the peri-wound skin at the ulcer margin (Eaglestein, 1993; Baxter, 2000).

Many dressings and topical treatments contain allergens that can result in inflammation (ie. allergic response). These local reactions can be uncomfortable, often resulting in itch or pain. Products with a high sensitisation potential (neomycin, bacitracin, lanolin, perfumes and natural rubber derivatives) should be avoided, particularly on patients with venous leg ulcers, where the sensitisation potential is greatest (_Chapter 6_) (Siegel, 2000).

Wound pain from inappropriate local wound care can generally be corrected by substituting a well thought-out local wound care regimen. The elements to remember include the use of dressings appropriate for moisture balance, bacterial balance, controlled inflammation, and autolytic debridement. This wound care regimen should be patient, wound, and disease specific.

Moisture balance

The dressing removal procedure is frequently cited by patients as the time they experience the greatest amount of pain (Hollinworth, 2000;

Puntillo *et al*, 2001; Kammerlander and Eberlein 2002; Sanders, 2002; Fauerbach *et al*, 2002; King, 2003). Pain at dressing change can be minimised by adopting strategies to reduce pain and trauma, and by choosing dressings with pain-reducing characteristics.

Some strategies to avoid pain with dressing changes include: soaking dressings with saline or even 4% topical lidocaine preparations, amethocaine 4% gel or EMLA prior to removal; using non-adhesive/ non-adherent dressings; or using atraumatic dressing products (eg. soft silicones). Many patients fear pain with dressing removal, so talking to the patient about their fears or concerns prior to the event is important. Having a plan for pain management in place prior to dressing changes helps to alleviate discomfort and anxiety. In addition, pain medications can be given an hour prior to dressing removal if pain is expected to occur.

Gauze dressings often stick to the wound and are painful. Soft silicone products have been recommended to help minimise pain and trauma on dressing removal (Hollinworth, 2000; Naylor, 2001). Hydrogels and alginates may also minimise pain in patients with mild to moderate exudate.

As with debridement, spinal cord injured patients may also experience pain and/or autonomic dysreflexia with dressing changes. These issues should also be addressed in this patient population.

Venous and leg ulcer pain

Treat the cause

Venous leg ulcers are the most common leg ulcers and increase in frequency with advancing age (Margolis *et al*, 2002). Although, historically, venous ulcers were thought to be relatively pain free, a significant number of patients with venous ulcers will experience pain that impacts on their quality of life (Phillips, 1994; Ryan *et al*, 2003; *Chapter 7*). Patients may have pain in the absence of an ulcer, and may experience prolonged pain once an ulcer has healed due to the other components of the underlying venous disease.

Venous disease consists of a spectrum of changes that slowly evolve over time. A variety of pain symptoms are associated. These range from discomfort and aching to deep, chronic pain. Acute, disabling pain may develop at each stage, and will impact on the plan of care for the patient (*Figure 8.2*).

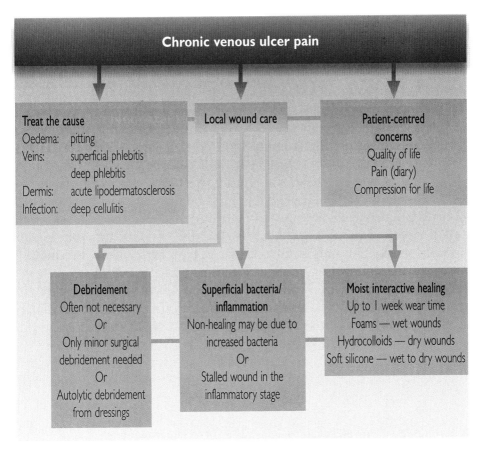

Figure 8.2: Venous ulcer pain paradigm (Ryan *et al*, 2003)

Patients with early stages of venous disease (ie. pitting oedema and prominent varicose veins) will often describe a dull aching or heaviness in their legs that worsens towards the end of the day, or after prolonged periods of standing as the oedema or fluid accumulation is maximal towards the end of the day. Support stockings, walking, and leg elevation while sitting will often relieve these symptoms. Attention must also be paid to other factors contributing to their venous stasis disease, such as obesity, sedentary lifestyle and other co-morbid illnesses. Once venous ulcers have healed, oedema control is essential for pain control and patients are advised to wear support stockings for life to control the oedema and prevent recurrence of ulcers.

Co-existing arterial disease must be ruled out, either clinically or by Doppler measurement of the ankle brachial pressure index (ABPI). Use of inappropriate compression bandaging in a patient with arterial insufficiency can lead to worsening of the ulcer and more serious complications. Ulcers related to arterial vascular disease have been traditionally considered to be painful; however, this feature alone is not adequate to differentiate a venous stasis ulcer from an ulcer resulting from arterial disease.

Long-standing pitting oedema leads to pigmentary changes, related to deposition of haemosiderin from extravasated red blood cells on the distal one-third to one-half of the legs. Over time, this pigmented area becomes sclerotic due to the leakage of fibrin. Lipodermatosclerosis consists of the triad of non-pitting oedema, sclerosis, and pigmentation. Pain is found in up to 43% of patients with lipodermatosclerosis, even without ulceration (Bruce, 2002). Lipodermatosclerosis may be further divided clinically into acute and chronic forms. The acute form consists of painful erythema mimicking an acute cellulitis with non-pitting oedema, in contrast to the chronic form, consisting of only sclerosis and pigmentation changes. Acute lipodermatosclerosis is sometimes mistaken for cellulitis, especially if it is unilateral. However, venous stasis changes are rarely unilateral, though the disease may have some asymmetry in terms of severity.

Management of lipodermatosclerosis includes: compression bandaging or support stockings; topical medications, including topical steroids and lubricants for skin surface erythema and dryness; and oral medication, including non-steroidal anti-inflammatory drugs (NSAIDs) (for pain), or pentoxifylline (for the woody fibrosis).

Support stockings may be adequate to control the symptoms of lipodermatosclerosis; however, non-steroidal anti-inflammatory medications may be needed for both their analgesic and anti-inflammatory properties. Adverse effects to this class of drugs must, of course, be considered prior to their use, particularly in the elderly (gastrointestinal haemorrhage, decreased renal function and increased cardiovascular risk).

Superficial or deep phlebitis must also be considered when patients describe a new pain or a change in pre-existing pain. Superficial phlebitis tends to present as 'bruise-like' pain over a localised portion of an inflamed and tender vein. The pain is often aggravated by palpation or standing, and the involved area may be quite warm to touch. The long saphenous vein is the vein most commonly involved.

Treatment options for superficial thrombophlebitis include

compression, walking and NSAID therapy. The role of the newer Cox-2 inhibitors has not yet been established in the management of superficial phlebitis. When patients with superficial thrombophlebitis are screened, an association with deep vein thrombosis is uncommon and it is unnecessary to look for the latter unless other risk factors are present (Bounameaux and Reber-Wasem, 1997).

Another factor that complicates venous disease and venous ulcers is the presence of dermatitis, particularly if it surrounds the wound (Reichert-Penetrat *et al*, 1999; Patel *et al*, 2001). Therefore, products used on the distal legs of patients with venous stasis must be relatively free of potential contact allergens and irritants (Wilson *et al*, 1991). Adhesives, tulles or paraffin gauze, topical lubricants and emollients, topical antibiotics, and other wound and peri-wound products all contain agents that can lead to contact dermatitis (Osmundswen, 1982; Floyer and Wilkinson, 1988; Zaki *et al*, 1994; Lopez Saez *et al*, 1998; Gooptu and Powell, 1999; Dong *et al*, 2002). Patients will complain of burning and itching, usually in the area of product application. Discomfort in association with eczematous changes, or a change in the type of pain, suggests irritation or allergic contact dermatitis (Anderson and Rajagopalan, 2001).

Atrophie blanche is one of the end stages of venous disease and consists of distinct white, sometimes star-shaped, depressed scar-like areas (Shornick *et al*, 1983). It is felt to develop spontaneously and is frequently associated with severe, sharp pain. Management of atrophie blanche pain can be challenging, and may require systemic analgesic medication.

The approach to venous ulcer pain must include an assessment of the cause of pain and the pain characteristics (constant or intermittent). Treatment can be local (eg. dressings, topical anaesthetic agents), regional (support rather than compression bandaging), or systemic (NSAIDs or other intermittent or long-acting pain medications).

Table 8.1: Differential diagnosis of venous pain

Diagnosis	Clinical/investigation	Treatment	Comments
Pitting oedema	Dull ache at end of day. Press thumb into skin and note degree of depression Grade 1+ to 4+	Compression bandaging, support stockings, walking, exercise. Improve calf muscle pump	Non-elastic stockings or compression bandaging may initially be preferred as they are less likely to cause pain at rest
Superficial phlebitis	Pain and tenderness along affected vein — usually saphenous	Compression, ambulation, NSAID therapy	Risk of associated underlying DVT is low, especially if affected area is below the knee
Deep vein thrombosis (DVT)	Acute, red, tender, swollen calf — almost too painful to touch. Doppler necessary to confirm diagnosis	ASA, unfractionated heparin, warfarin Low-molecular weight heparin Bed rest	Suspect a DVT in patients with a sudden increase in calf pain, with risk factors such as immobilisation, recent surgery, oral contraceptives, etc
Acute lipodermato-sclerosis	Diffuse, purple-red swollen leg resembling cellulitis, aching and tenderness is common	Compression bandaging, support stockings, NSAIDs	Usually bilateral, although may be more prominent on one leg. Compression therapy essential
Chronic lipodermato-sclerosis	Diffuse, brown sclerotic pigmentation with widespread chronic pain	Same as with acute lipodermatosclerosis, but with topical steroids and lubricants. Pentoxifylline	Support stockings may have to be custom made to accommodate for leg shape
Wound infection	Change in pain character associated with other clinical signs of infection	Topical antimicrobial agents and oral antibiotics, if indicated	Maintain bacterial balance, and watch for increase in pain, size, exudate, odour or changes in granulation tissue as signs of infection
Cellulitis	Diffuse, bright red, hot leg, usually unilateral, associated with tenderness and often fever	Oral antibiotics, with IV antibiotics needed for severe episodes or with low host resistance	Venous ulcers may make individuals more prone to cellulitis
Atrophie blanche	Pain, stellate, white scar-like areas associated with pain at rest and standing	NSAID therapy Other analgesics	May be seen in association with scars of healed ulcers, or may be an independent clinical feature
Acute contact dermatitis	Itching, burning red areas on leg corresponding to area of use of topical product	Remove the allergen Apply topical steroids	Lanolin, colophony, latex, neomycin are some of the more likely agents involved

Patient-centred concerns

Although venous ulcers have historically been described as painless, it is now known that a significant number of patients with venous ulcers will experience pain that impacts on their quality of life (Krasner, 1998).

Local wound care

There are many ways to debride a venous ulcer. Sharp surgical debridement is often not necessary and when performed may be quite painful. Topical anaesthetics, such as topical xylocaine (1–4%) preparations, EMLA or amethocaine 4% gel have been used clinically in appropriate settings prior to debridement to improve pain (Lok, 1999). Autolytic debriding agents are useful, particularly hydrogels or hydrocolloids, and may actually help reduce the pain. Mechanical debridement using wet-to-dry dressings is generally too painful to be tolerated, and more beneficial alternatives exist. Enzymatic debriding agents can be used for thick adherent eschar as an alternative to hydrocolloids or hydrogels.

Diabetic foot ulcer pain

Treat the cause

Persons with diabetic foot ulcers require not only adequate vasculature and infection control, but also pressure downloading or redistribution.

In contrast to ischaemic pain, diabetic neuropathic pain is not generally associated with increased activity, but often appears during periods of diminished external sensory stimulation (eg. at night). Because of its multifactorial nature, no single treatment has proven a panacea (Jensen and Larson, 2001; Simmons and Feldman, 2002). Neuropathic pain often responds incompletely to traditional anti-inflammatory and opioid pain medication (Gilron *et al*, 2005).

Tricyclic antidepressants have been used successfully, especially for treatment of burning pain. Second generation tricyclics with high noradrenaline activity, such as nortriptylene or desipramine, are often the preferred choices. Newer anti-epileptic drugs, such as gabapentin or pregabulin, have also been used with success.

Although neuropathic pain may occur in these patients, pain is not common in the diabetic foot ulcer itself. When ulcer pain does occur, it may herald the onset of limb-threatening complications such as critical ischaemia, deep infection, or Charcot arthropathy.

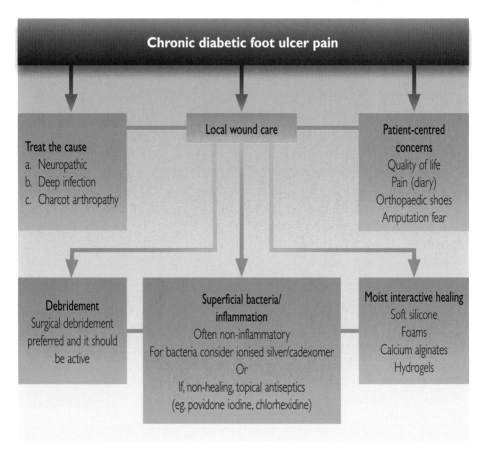

Figure 8.3: Diabetic foot ulcer pain paradigm (Sibbald *et al*, 2003)

Critical ischaemia

Pulses are generally palpable in the foot with around 80 mmHg systolic pressure in the dorsalis pedis artery. In patients with diabetes and in elderly patients without diabetes, the ankle brachial pressure index (ABPI) may be falsely high because of calcified arteries. Therefore, further non-invasive tests, such as toe pressure or transcutaneous oxygen pressure, are necessary. Toe pressure over 50 mmHg, or transcutaneous oxygen pressure over 300 mmHg, are usually required to ensure sustained healing. In extreme cases, ischaemia can cause pain at rest. These patients require a consultation with a vascular surgeon for possible surgical reconstruction or arterial dilation to improve flow (Gibbons *et al*, 1993; Akbari and LoGerfo, 1999; Akbari *et al*, 2000).

Deep infection

Wound infections, particularly those involving deep plantar spaces, can cause pain even in the presence of severe neuropathy. Unfortunately, this pain is often overlooked since signs and symptoms of infection in the person with diabetes are often subtle. The presence of non-neuropathic pain in even a mildly erythematous or oedematous diabetic foot, even with a normal X-ray of the foot, requires assessment and, if necessary, treatment (Sibbald *et al*, 2003a). Peri-ulcer erythema greater than 2 cm represents limb-threatening changes (Caputo *et al*, 1997). Patients may have new areas of breakdown and ulcer enlargement as their only indicators of deep infection. The extension or probing of the ulcer to bone, in concert with serial radiography or magnetic resonance imaging (MRI), may be an effective means to evaluate the potential extent of bony involvement and osteomyelitis (Grayson *et al*, 1995; Tomas *et al*, 2000).

Charcot arthropathy

Charcot arthropathy is characterised by pathologic fractures, joint dislocation and foot deformity in patients with severe neuropathy (Sanders and Frykberg, 1991; Sanders and Frykberg, 1993; Armstrong *et al*; 1997; Armstrong and Lavery, 1998), and is aggravated by weight bearing. Pain is the presenting complaint in 75% of cases, along with a red, hot, swollen foot. The treatment of Charcot arthropathy requires pressure downloading or offloading until the skin surface temperature becomes normal (Armstrong and Lavery, 1997).

Patient-centred concerns

Pain in the neuropathic foot often reflects a deep infection or acute Charcot arthropathy, and places the patient at higher risk for amputation. Detection of diabetic foot problems often occurs late, and the human and economic cost of diabetic foot ulcers and amputation remains high (Wishner and Rubin, 2001). Individuals with diabetes need to be informed about the risks and complications, understand the loss of protective sensation (LOPS), and be taught the problem-solving skills necessary to respond to health-related problems. Dressings and pressure offloading devices are often expensive and the healthcare professional may need to consult with appropriate agencies to facilitate access to such treatments for their patients.

Local wound care

Debridement is usually painless due to underlying neuropathy. If pain is present, ischaemia, deep infection or Charcot arthropathy should be considered. Although sharp surgical debridement is the procedure of choice (Steed, 1995), it should only be performed when blood supply is adequate for healing. Debridement should include removal of callus and friable bright red or exuberant granulation. Calcium alginate dressings post debridement will help control surface bleeding and prevent the formation of a haemorrhagic crust. Autolytic mechanical and enzymatic debridement are less effective.

Superficial infection may cause local pain or discomfort due to the release of pre-inflammatory mediators by the bacteria and the host, but it is much more likely that pain is indicative of infection in the deeper compartment. Signs and symptoms of increased bacterial burden have been reviewed with the mnemonic NERDS for superficial compartment increased bacterial burden, and STONES for the deep or surrounding skin infection.

Some patients with diabetes may have decreased inflammatory response that delays healing, particularly with poor diabetic control and a high gycosylated haemoglobin value. All persons with diabetes have a relative immune deficiency that decreases host resistance and results in an increased damage from the effect of bacteria within the chronic wound.

Table 8.2: Diabetic foot ulcer pain

Neuropathic	Charcot foot	Deep infection
Neuropathic pain is due to irritation or damage of the nerve fibres	Recurrent minor trauma (not perceived due to neuropathy)	Deep infection needs to be distinguished from superficial infection. The following signs and symptoms are often useful.
There are 3 components to the neuropathy:	→ Minor fractures	**Superficial** (try topical treatment x 2 weeks) • Non-healing • ↑ Exudate • Bright red granulation • Friable exuberant granulation • New areas of slough
Sensory — test with monofilaments ↓ sensation **Autonomic** — check for dry skin (DDx tinea) **Motor** — ↓ reflexes, claw toes	→ Continuous trauma results in disintegration	**Deep** (need systemic treatment) • Pain • New areas of breakdown • Dermal erythema >2cm • Warmth • Probe to bone
Nerve irritation often causes burning (try tricyclics)	→ Contact cast (or other off-loading) →	
Nerve damage often causes shooting or stabbing pain. Often tricyclics are not successful and gabapentin may be the treatment of choice	*Monitor:* Swelling Warmth (skin temp) Biochemical markers of bone formation	

Excess moisture in diabetic foot ulcers leads to macerated callus around the edge of the wound edge and may favour bacterial proliferation (Edmonds, 2006). This often results in increased pain. Moisture control is therefore crucial, and best achieved through moisture absorptive dressings, such as foams, Hydrofiber®, and calcium alginates, along with callus debridement. If the wound edges are macerated, protection around the outer rim can be accomplished through application of zinc oxide paste, petrolatum, film-forming liquid acrylates, windowed hydrocolloid or film dressings (Romanelli et al, 2003).

Pressure ulcer pain

Treat the cause

Pain is the end result of tissue damage and pressure ulcer formation, but the pain may also contribute to further immobility. Spinal cord injured, elderly, and cognitively-impaired patients with pressure ulcers present special challenges in pain management. Up to 80% of nursing home residents with pressure ulcers have significant pain that is under treated (American Geriatrics Society [AGS], 2002; Reddy et al, 2003a). Although age alone is not a risk factor for increased pain, age has been identified as a key risk factor for inadequate pain management (Cobbs et al, 1999; AGS, 2002).

Pressure ulcers develop from unrelieved pressure, often over bony prominences. This pressure often exceeds capillary closing pressure, resulting in tissue ischaemia. Tissue ischaemia itself leads to pain through the release of inflammatory mediators. Pressure relief and reduction provided by support surfaces are components in the treatment of the cause of the ulcers. These surfaces often off-load pressure from bony prominences, but they may also aid in pain management. Seating and positioning assessments by trained professionals are an important part of pain management in persons with pressure ulcers. All institutionalised patients should be on pressure reduction foam mattresses and seating surfaces to prevent pressure ulcers and to provide comfort.

Nutritional support is also important in pressure ulcer healing and pain management. Healing of pressure ulcers is compromised by moisture from incontinence of stools and urine, friction and shear, decreased mobility and poor nutritional status (Green *et al*, 1999; Cunha *et al*, 2000; Thomas, 2001). Poor nutrition leads to decreased muscle mass and wasting of protective subcutaneous fat, and patients with significant muscle wasting tend to experience greater pain. Nutritional demands for protein and calorie intake are actually greater in patients with pressure ulcers, and nutritional consultation is important for optimal management (Russell, 2001; Westergren *et al*, 2001; Todorovic, 2002).

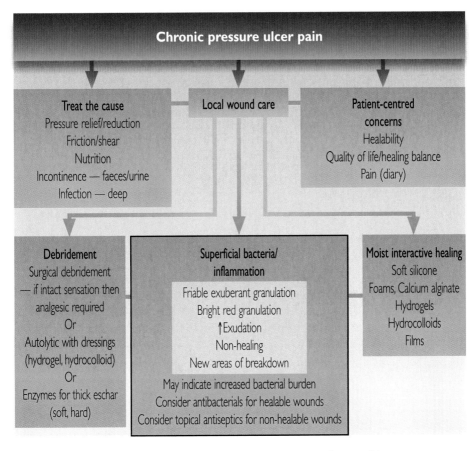

Figure 8.4: Pressure ulcer pain paradigm (Reddy *et al*, 2003b)

Pressure ulcers may also cause damage or irritation to peripheral nerves, leading to neuropathic pain. The burning pain of nerve irritation may respond to tricyclic antidepressants, while the stabbing pain of nerve damage may require anticonvulsants, such as gabapentin or pregabulin.

Table 8.3: Pressure ulcer pain management strategies

Cause of pain	Definition	Treatment	Comments
Pressure	A force applied to the skin and underlying tissues which inhibits blood flow when it ↓ pressures within the capillary Capillary closing pressure (CCP) = 32 mmHg (average value)	Special surface: Pressure reduction: ↓ pressure, but not necessarily below CCP eg. high density foam, standard hospital mattresses synthetic (not sheepskin heel booties Pressure relief: ↓ pressure below CCP eg. dynamic flow beds, turning schedules crucial	Consider: Pressure mapping Wheelchair assessment
Friction	Created by movement of the patient over a surface	Heel booties, eg. sheepskin booties (do not reduce pressure but may decrease friction) Careful with patient transfers (use turning sheet) Hydrocolloid over bony prominences	On its own, friction does not usually cause ulcers. However, friction in addition to pressure greatly increases risk of ulcer development
Shear	Adjacent body surfaces slide across each other (as happens when a patient slides down a bed)	Keep head of bed ≤ 30 degrees Tilt seating, rather than recline (may need some recline if slumping is a problem)	Again, more dangerous when combined with pressure
Moisture	Irritation and maceration from sweating, stool, urine, wound drainage	Prevention: If urine incontinence — bladder training; urinary catheter (in and out rather than permanent, if possible) Change undergarment pads frequently Local wound care to keep surrounding skin from maceration Absorbent surface next to skin Treatment Barriers to wound edge (eg. zinc oxide, petrolatum, occlusive dressings) May need anti-diarrhoea medications If surrounding dermatitis, may need steroid cream/ointment	Can also use film-forming topical acrylate liquids Watch for secondary yeast, especially in folds

Table 8.3: Cont

Cause of pain	Definition	Treatment	Comments
Peri-ulcer irritation	Can be due to dermatitis, maceration, and/or infection (eg. candida)	To reduce peri-ulcer irritation apply either vaseline, zinc oxide, film-forming liquid (eg. acrylate), occlusive dressings (picture frame technique) and, if candida suspected, hydrocortisone in canestan cream, twice daily	If hydrocortisone in canestan is being easily wiped off with body positioning and movement, then cover with zinc oxide
Nutrition	Both pain and healing may be exacerbated if a patient has low muscle mass	Major risks: low overall dietary intake, especially protein Consult dietician Consider supplements	No particular evidence that certain vitamins promote healing Check albumin and total lymphocyte count
Deep infection	Infection requiring systemic agents	Probe to bone — osteomyleitis unless proven otherwise, may need long-term antibiotics	Probe ulcer. Make sure it does not probe to bone and there are no sinus tracts or fistulas
Neuropathic/radicular	Nerve irritation, damage	Consider tricyclic antidepressants (nortryptiline), anticonvulsants (gabapentin)	Consider referral to anaesthesia for nerve blocks
Spasms	Involuntary muscle movement	May need baclofen	Consider referral to psychiatry

Regrettably, paralysis does not mean freedom from pain. Patients with spinal cord injuries may experience spasms, leading to damaging friction and shear in locations such as the heels, which may result in skin breakdown. The anti-spasmotic, baclofen, can be used to help control spasms; however, a referral to a specialist in physical medicine and rehabilitation may be beneficial for optimal patient care.

Patient-centred concerns

The patient and healthcare professional should work together to define common goals of care, and to define their respective roles and responsibilities in the therapeutic relationship. Persons with pressure ulcers and healthcare professionals may decide that it is not reasonable to set healing as a goal for the patient, given declining health status or other related factors, such as treatment side-effects and availability. Instead, the focus may be on pain control, management of infection, exudate, odour, and improved quality of life. Non-healable wounds may require the use of topical antiseptics with low tissue toxicity and sensitisation potential.

Local wound care

Severely demented patients who are bed-bound and develop pressure ulcers still feel pain with debridement, although they may not be able to effectively communicate their discomfort. It is important to use simple pain assessment scales (such as a faces tool), or to watch for non-verbal pain clues, such as agitation or facial grimacing. As previously discussed, patients with paralysis may still experience pain with debridement. It is important to discuss any unpleasant experience with each patient, as sensations differ between individuals. Some patients with spinal cord paralysis will require local anaesthetic prior to debridement to prevent autonomic dysreflexia. Severe muscle spasms with previous interventions are a clue that local anaesthetic use may be beneficial.

Conclusion

Pain is what the patient says it is. Optimal patient care must combine environmental and non-pharmacological interventions with appropriate pharmacological interventions, through an appropriate analysis of patient-centred concerns (Jacox *et al*, 1994; Ferrell, 1996). Assessment of pain must include the treatment of the cause and in this chapter we have discussed venous, diabetic foot and pressure ulcer related diagnoses and treatment. Local wound care may be slightly different in the three different causes of chronic wounds, but they all must consider tissue debridement, superficial increased bacterial burden or prolonged inflammation and moisture balance as components of optimal wound bed preparation. A painful, chronic wound often indicates that there is something wrong and it needs to be corrected. Patients need to be empowered to discuss pain with healthcare professionals in a non-threatening environment of co-operation. Advanced knowledge of the principles of pain management for healthcare professionals needs to be coupled with the ability to prescribe the appropriate pharmacological agents, and an interprofessional team to optimise care. By listening to the patient's perspective, optimal wound and pain management can be combined with successful outcomes. Even though ulcer healing is not always possible, we can improve the activities of daily living and quality of life of most of our patients.

References

Akbari CM, LoGerfo FW (1999) Diabetes and peripheral vascular disease. *J Vasc Surg* 30(2): 373–84

Akbari CM, Pomposelli FB, Gibbons GW *et al* (2000) Lower extremity revascularization in diabetes: late observations. *Arch Surg* 135(4): 452–6

American Geriatrics Society Panel on Persistent Pain in Older Persons (2002) The management of persistent pain in older persons. *J Am Geriatr Soc* 50: S205–S224

Anderson RT, Rajagopalan R (2001) Effects of allergic dermatosis on health related quality of life. *Curr Allergy Asthma Rep* 1(4): 309–15

Armstrong DG, Lavery LA (1997) Montiroing healing of acute Charcot's arthropathy with infrared dermal thermometry. *J Rehabil Res Dev* 34(3): 317–21

Armstrong DG, Lavery LA (1998) Acute Charcot's arthropathy of the foot and ankle. *Phys Ther* 78: 74–80

Armstrong DG, Todd WF, Lavery LA, Harkless LB (1997) The natural history of acute Charcot's arthropathy in a diabetic foot specialty clinic. *Diabetic Med* 14: 357–63

Baxter H (2000) A comparison of two hydrocolloid sheet dressings. *Br J Community Nurs* 5(11): 572–7

Bowler PG (2002) Wound pathophysiology, infection and therapeutic options. *Ann Med* 34(6): 419–27

Bowler PG (2003) Bacterial growth guideline: reassessing its clinical relevance in wound healing. *Ostomy/Wound Management* 49(1): 44–53

Bounameaux H, Reber-Wasem MA (1997) Superficial thrombophlebitis and deep vein thrombosis. A controversial association. *Arch Intern Med* 157(16): 1822–4

Bruce AJ *et al* (2002) Lipodermatosclerosis: Review of cases evaluated at Mayo Clinic. *J Am Acad Dermatol* 46: 187–92

Caputo GM, Joshi N, Weitekamp MR (1997) Foot infections in patients with diabetes. *Am Fam Physician* 56(1): 195–202

Cobbs E *et al* (1999) *Geriatrics Review Syllabus: A Core Curriculum in Geriatric Medicine.* 4th edn. American Geriatrics Society

Cunha DF, Frota RB, Arruda MS, Cunha SF, Teixeira VP (2000) Pressure sores among malnourished necropsied adults-preliminary data. *Rev Hosp Clin Fac Med Sao Paulo* 55(3): 79–82

Davies CE, Turton G, Woolfrey G, ElleyR, Taylor M (2005) Exploring debridement options for chronic venous leg ulcers. *Br J Nurs* 14(7); 393–7

Dong H, Kerl H, Cerroni L (2002) EMLA cream induced irritant contact dermatitis. *J Cutan Pathol* 29(3): 190–2

Eager CA (2005) Dressings and clinician support in relieving pain and promoting healing. *Ostomy/Wound Managment* 51(8): 12–14

Eaglestein WH (1993) Occlusive dressings. *J Dermatol Surg Oncol* 19(8): 716–20

Edmonds M (2006) Diabetic foot ulcers: practical treatment recommendations. *Drugs* 66(7): 913–29

Fauerbach JA, Lawrence JW, Haythornthwaite JA, Richter L (2002) Coping with the stress of a painful medical procedure. *Behav Res Ther* 40(9): 1003–15

Ferrell BR (1996) Patient education and non-drug interventions. In: Ferrell BR, Ferrell BA, eds. *Pain in the Elderly.* IASP Press, Seattle: 35–44

Fletcher J (2005) Understanding wound dressings: hydrocolloids. *Nurs Times* **101**(46): 51

Floyer C, Wilkinson JD (1988) Treatment of venous leg ulcers with cadexomer iodine with particular reference to iodine sensitivity. *Acta Chir Scand* Suppl **544**: 60–1

Gardner SE, Frantz RA, Troia C, Eastman S, MacDonal M, Buresh K, Healy D (2001) A tool to assess clinical sign and symptoms of localized infection in chronic wounds: development and reliability. *Ostomy/Wound Management* **47**(1): 40–7

Gibbons GW, Marcaccio EJJ, Burgess AM *et al* (1993) Improved quality of diabetic foot care, 1984 vs. 1990: reduced length of stay and costs, insufficient reimbursement. *Arch Surg* **128**: 576–81

Gilron I, Bailey JM, Tu D, Holden RR, Weaver DF, Houlden RL (2005) Morphine, gabapentin, or their combination for neuropathic pain. *N Engl J Med* **352**(13): 1324–34

Gniadecka M *et al* (1998) Removal of dermal edema with class I and II compression stockings in patients with lipodermatosclerosis. *J Am Acad Dermatol* **39**: 966–70

Gooptu C, Powell SM (1999) The problems of rubber hypersensitivity (Types I and IV) in chronic leg ulcer and stasis eczema patients. *Contact Dermatitis* **41**(2): 89–93

Green SM, Winterberg H, Franks PJ, Moffatt CJ, Eberhardie C, McLaren S (1999) Nutritional intake in community patients with pressure ulcers. *J Wound Care* **8**(7): 325–30

Helme RD, Gibson SJ (1999) Pain in older people. In: Crombie IK, Croft PR, Linton SJ *et al*, eds. *Epidemiology of Pain.* IASP Press, Seattle: 103–12

Hollingworth H (2000) Pain and wound care. Wound Care Society Educational Leaflet. *Wound Care Society* **7**(2)

Hollinworth H, Collier M (2000) Nurses' views about pain and trauma at dressing changes: results of a national survey. *J Wound Care* **9**(8): 369–73

Jacox A, Carr DB, Payne R *et al* (1994) Management of cancer pain. Clinical Practice Guideline No 9. AHCPR Publication No 94-0592. Rockville, MD: Agency for Health Care Policy and Research, US. Department of Health and Human Services, Public Health Service

Jensen PG, Larson JR (2001) Management of painful diabetic neuropathy. *Drugs Aging* **18**(10): 737–49

Kammerlander G, Eberlein T (2002) Nurses' views about pain and trauma at dressing changes: a central European perspective. *J Wound Care* **11**(2): 76–9

Kannon GA, Garrett AB (1995) Moist wound healing with occlusive dressings. A clinical review. *Dermatol Surg* **21**(7): 583–90

King B (2003) Pain at first dressing change after toenail avulsion: the experience of nurses, patients and an observer: 1. *J Wound Care* **12**(1): 5–10

Krasner D (1998) Painful venous ulcers: themes and stories about their impact on quality of life. *Ostomy/Wound Management* **44**(9): 38–49

Krasner D, Sibbald RG (1999) Local aspects of diabetic foot ulcer care: assessment, dressings and topical agents. In: Levin ME, O'Neal DN, Bowker JH, eds. *The Diabetic Foot*. 6th edn. Mosby-Yearbook, St Louis

Lok C *et al* (1999) EMLA cream as a topical anesthetic for the repeated mechanical debridement of venous leg ulcers: A double-blind, placebo-controlled study. *J Am Acad Dermatol* **40**: 208–13

Lopez Saez MP, de Barrio M, Zubeldia JM, Prieto A, Olalde S, Baeza ML (1998) Acute IgE-mediated generalized urticaria-angiedema after topical application of povidone-iodine. *Allergol Immunopathol (Madr)* **26**(1): 23–6

Margolis D, Bilker W, Santanna J, Baumgarten M (2002) Venous leg ulcer: Incidence and prevalence in the elderly. *J Am Acad Dermatolol* **46**(3): 381–6

Mast BA, Schultz GS (1996) Interactions of cytokines, growth factors, and proteases in acute and chronic wounds. *Wound Rep Regen* **4**: 411–20

Meuleneire F (2002) Using a soft silicone-coated net dressing to manage skin tears. *J Wound Care* **11**(10): 365–9

Naylor W (2001) Assessment and management of pain in fungating wounds. *Br J Nurs* **10**(22)(Suppl): S53–S52

Neil JA, Munjas BA (2000) Living with a chronic wound: the voices of sufferers. *Ostomy/Wound Management* **46**(5): 28–38

Osmundsen PE (1982) Contact dermatitis to chlorhexidine. *Contact Dermatitis* **8**(2): 81–3

Patel GK, Llewellyn M, Harding KG (2001) Managing gravitational eczema and allergic contact dermatitis. *Br J Community Nurs* **6**(8): 394–406

Phillips T, Stanton B, Provan A, Lew R (1994) A study of the impact of leg ulcers on quality of life: financial, social, and psychologic implications. *J Am Acad Dermatol* **31**(1): 49–53

Puntillo KA, White C, Morris AB, Perdue ST, Stanik-Hutt J, Thompson CL, Wild LR (2001) Patients' perceptions and responses to procedural pain: results from Thunder Project II. *Am J Crit Care* **10**(4): 238–51

Queen D, Woo K, Schulz VN, Sibbald RG (2005) Chronic wound pain and palliative cancer care. *Ostomy/Wound Management* **51**(11A Suppl): 9–11

Reddy M, Keast D, Fowler E, Sibbald RG (2003a) Pain in pressure ulcers. *Ostomy/Wound Management* **49**(4 Suppl): 30–5

Reddy M, Kohr R, Queen D, Keast D, Sibbald RG (2003b) Practical treatment of wound pain and trauma: a patient-centered approach. An overview. *Ostomy/Wound Management* **49**(4 Suppl): 2–15

Reichert-Penetrat S, Barbaud A, Weber M, Schmutz JL (1999) Leg ulcers. Allergologic studies of 359 cases. *Ann Dermatol Venereol* **126**(2): 131–5

Romanelli M, Looverbosch D, Heyman H, Meaume S, Ciangherotti, Charpin S (2003) An open multi-center randonmised study comparing a sef-adherent soft silicone foam dressing versus a hydropolymer dressing, in patients with pressure ulcer stage II according to the EPUAP guidelines. Poster Presentation, EWMA meeting 2002

Rovee DT (1991) Evolution of wound dressings and their effects on the healing process. *Clin Mater* **8**(3–4): 183–8

Russell L (2001) The importance of patients' nutritional status in wound healing. *Br J Nurs* **10**(6 Suppl):S42, S44–S49

Ryan S, Eager C, Sibbald RG (2003) Venous leg ulcer pain. *Ostomy/Wound Management* **49**(4 Suppl): 16–-23

Sanders LJ, Frykberg RG (1991) The Charcot foot. In: Frykberg, ed. *The High Risk Foot in Diabetes Mellitus*. Churchill Livingstone, New York: 325–35

Sanders LJ, Frykberg RG (1993) Charcot's Joint. In: Levin ME, O'Neal LW Bowker JH, eds. *The Diabetic Foot*. 2nd edn. Mosby-Year Book, St Louis

Sanders C (2002) A review of current practice for boys undergoing hypospdias repair: from pre-operative work up to removal of dressing post surgery. *J Child Health Care* **6**(1): 60–9

Shornick JK, Nicholes BK, Bergstresser PR, Gilliam JN (1983) Idiopathic atrophie blanche. *J Am Acad Dermatol* **8**(6): 792–8

Sibbald RG (1998) Venous leg ulcers. *Ostomy/Wound Management* **44**(9): 52–64

Sibbald RG (2003) Topical antimicrobials. Ostomy/Wound Management **49**(5A Suppl): 14–8

Sibbald RG, Williamson D, Orsted HL, Campbell K, Keast D, Krasner D, Sibbald D (2000) Preparing the wound bed — debridement, bacterial balance and moisture balance. *Ostomy/Wound Management* **46**(11): 14–22, 24–8, 30–5

Sibbald RG, Armstrong DG, Orsted HL (2003a) Pain in diabetic foot ulcers. *Ostomy/Wound Management* **49**(4 Suppl): 24–9

Sibbald RG, Orsted H, Schultz GS, Coutts P, Keast D (2003b) International Wound Bed Preparation Advisory Board; Canadian Chronic Wound Advisory Board. Preparing the wound bed 2003: focus on infection and inflammation. *Ostomy/Wound Management* **49**(11): 23–51

Siegel DM (2000) Contact sensitivity and recalcitrant wounds. *Ostomy/Wound Management* **46**(1A Suppl): 65S–74S

Simmons Z, Feldman EL (2002) Update on diabetic neuropathy. *Curr Opin Neurol* **15**(5): 595–603

Sinha S, Munichoodapa CS, Kozak GP (1972) Neuroarthropathy (Charcot joints) in diabetes mellitus. *Medicine* **51**: 191–210

Steed DL (1995) Diabetic Ulcer Study Group. Clinical evaluation of recombinant human platelet-derived growth factor for the treatment of lower extremity diabetic ulcers. *J Vasc Surg* **21**: 71–81

Thomas DR (2001) Improving outcome of pressure ulcers with nutritional interventions: a review of the evidence. *Nutrition* **17**(2): 121–5

Tomas MB, Patel M, Marwin SE, Palestro CJ (2000) The diabetic foot. *Br J Radiol* **73**(868): 443–50

Todorovic V (2002) Food and wounds: nutritional factors in wound formation and healing. *Br J Community Nurs* Sept: 43–4, 46, 48

Weaver LC, Marsh DR, Gris D, Brown A, Dekaban GA (2006) Autonomic dysreflexia after spinal cord injury: central mechanisms and strategies for prevention. *Prog Brain Res* **152**: 245–63

Westergren A, Karlsson S, Andersson P, Ohlsson O, Hallberg IR (2001) Eating difficulties, need for assisted eating, nutritional status and pressure ulcers in patients admitted for stroke rehabilitation. *J Clin Nurs* **10**(2): 257–69

Wilson CL, Cameron J, Powell SM, Cherry G, Ryan TJ (1991) High incidence of contact dermatitis in leg-ulcer patients — implications for management. *Clin Exp Dermatol* **16**(4): 250–3

Wishner WJ, Rubin RR (2001) Empowerment in amputation prevention. In: Bowker JH, Pfeifer MA eds. *Levin and O'Neal's The Diabetic Foot*. 6th edn. Mosby, St Louis

World Union of Wound Healing Societies (2004) *Principles of Best Practice: Minimising pain at wound dressing-related procedures. A consensus document*. Available online at: www.wuwhs.org/pdf/consensus_eng.pdf

Wright JB, Lam K, Buret AG, Olson ME, Burrell RE (2002) Early healing events in a porcine model of contaminated wounds: effects of nanocrystalline silver on matrix metalloprotineases, cell apoptosis and healing. *Wound Rep Regen* **10**(3): 141–51

Zaki I, Shall L, Dalziel KL (1994) Bacitracin: a significant sensitizer in leg ulcer patients? *Contact Dermatitis* **31**(2): 92–4

Appendix: Pain management medications
(always follow the manufacturer's instructions carefully)

Class of medication	Examples	Starting doses	Comments
Antipyretics	Paracetamol (Acetaminophen)	Start 500 mg QID Max daily dose 4 × 1 g	Maximum dose in the elderly should be closer to 2 g/day
NSAIDs (non-steroidal anti-inflammatory drugs)	Ibuprofen Ketotophen	400 mg BID 50 mg OD	Consider adding GI protective agent if at higher risk of GI bleeding; if frail elderly, consider different class of agents due to high risk of bleeding
	Cox-II inhibitors Rofecoxib (Vioxx)	25 mg OD	
	Celecoxib (Celebrex)	100 mg BID	
Opioids S = short-acting L = long-acting	Codeine (S)	15–30 mg q4h PRN	Can increase dosage of long-acting every few days if requiring several short-acting (breakthrough) doses — watch for sedative side-effects
	Codeine Contin (L)	50 mg BID	
	Morphine (S)	2.5–5.0 mg q4h PRN	
	Morphine contin (L)	15 mg BID	
	Fentanyl (L) transdermal	1 × 25 µg/hr patch every 3 days	
	Oxycodone (S)	10 mg q4h PRN	
Adjuvant medications: Tricyclic anti-depressants	Nortriptyline or desipramine or amitryptyline	10 mg Nocte (increase as required to about 50 mg/day)	Add to a regimen of any of the above medications for possible synergistic benefit
Anti-epileptics	Gabapentin	300 mg OD (increase to TID, max dose 1800 mg/day)	Watch for anticholinergic side-effects (dry mouth, urinary incontinence, drowsiness, confusion) in the elderly
Anti-depressants	Carbamazepine	100 mg OD (increase to BID, max dose 1200 mg/day)	

Chapter 9

The psychology of pain and its application to wound management

Patricia Price

Pain is a sensation that, with a few rare exceptions, we all experience at some point in our lives. Many of us will remember falling over as a young child and the rituals that surrounded the experience, including having someone to 'kiss-it-better'. The universality of the pain experience is such that we can all relate in some way to those who live with pain all the time — although, fortunately, relatively few of us have first-hand experience of constant or severe pain. This chapter focuses on our changing understanding of the pain experience, and how theoretical perspectives have evolved to include the emotional component of pain. The chapter also deals with the psychological aspects of pain and pain management, then applies these principles to patients with wound-associated pain problems.

A little bit of history

There is historical evidence that ancient civilisations recorded on stone tablets how they treated those in pain, using treatments such as pressure, heat, water, and the power of the sun. The history of the dark ages shows that the treatment of pain was often left to sorcerers, witches and/or priests, who used herbs as part of elaborate ceremonies to drive away evil spirits and demons. Although there is some evidence that Greek and Roman civilisations understood that the brain had a role in the perception of pain, it was not until Leonardo da Vinci that the thinkers of the time understood that the brain was the central organ responsible for sensation, and that the spinal cord might play a key role.

During the 16th and 17th centuries, many philosophers debated the relationship between the body and the mind; the location of the 'mind' being a point of controversy (known as Cartesian Dualism). In 1664, René Descartes, who was particularly intrigued by the mind-body split, proposed a 'pain pathway' — a theoretical approach that dominated thinking about pain for almost two hundred and fifty years.

Descartes proposed that pain was a sensation that was the result of an external noxious stimulus (such as fire), which triggered a reaction in nerve filaments along a pathway that led directly to a centre in the brain which, in turn, triggered the sensation of pain. He used the example of ringing a bell to explain the concept: when you pull on the rope (stimulus), the vibration passes along the rope (activation of the nerve filaments), until the bell starts to ring (the message gets to the pain centre of the brain). His concept is clearly outlined in the famous illustration (*Figure 9.1*). Indeed, Descartes believed that the amount of pain felt was directly related to the severity of the stimulus: the greater the fire, the greater the pain.

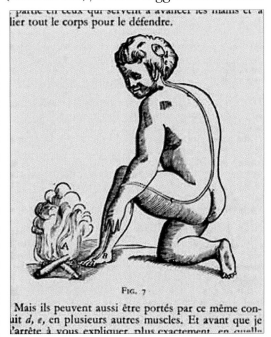

Figure 9.1: The pain pathway proposed by Descartes in 1664

For many years, this view of pain remained the recognised theory, but physicians and nurses became increasingly aware that not all types of pain experience fitted in with this perspective, particularly following the injuries suffered by soldiers during war. In 1895, Strong and others began to think of pain in a new way, and proposed that pain was actually due to two factors:

1. The sensation of pain.
2. The person's reaction to pain.

For the first time, psychological and organic causes were seen to be important (Brannon and Feist, 1997).

After the Second World War, evidence began to emerge that soldiers wounded in battle reported little pain, despite horrific injuries (Beecher, 1946). The explanation given was that having been taken away from the battle field and the threat of imminent death, the solders were in an optimistic frame of mind. Ten years later, this view was supported by a further study (Beecher, 1956), which reported that civilians injured during the war reported higher levels of pain and requested more pain relief than soldiers wounded in the Second World War, despite having less severe injuries. This led Beecher to conclude that, 'the intensity of suffering is largely determined by what the pain means to the patient' (1956).

At around the same time in the UK, a story hit the headlines that resulted in the general public becoming more aware of the complexity of the pain experience. In 1956, Bert Trautman played as goalkeeper in the FA Cup Final for the winning side Manchester City. However, in the 74th minute, he made a dramatic dive for the ball and sustained a severe neck injury. The pitch-side first-aid included a bucket of water and a sponge; so the 'magic' sponge was applied and Bert carried on playing. It was only after he collected his winner's medal that Bert began to complain of headaches — severe headaches. He was taken to the hospital where it was discovered that he had a broken neck. This story has become a football legend, but also serves to reflect a more modern understanding of pain. There are certain circumstances when pain does not necessarily pass into consciousness and can be denied.

Around the same time in the USA two researchers, Ronald Melzack and Peter Wall, were becoming interested in pain and in 1965 proposed a new theory. They believed that pain was not the result of a linear process that begins with a simulation of a pain pathway and ends with the experience of pain. They proposed that pain perception is subject to a number of modulations that can influence the experience of pain, and these modulations begin in the spinal cord. They (1965) hypothesised that structures in the spinal cord act as a gate for the sensory input that is interpreted as pain: neural mechanisms in the spinal cord can either increase the flow of information (and open the gate to increased sensation), or decrease the flow of neural impulses (and close the gate). The theory became known as the 'gate control theory' (GCT).

In later years, Melzack and Wall (1982, 1988) pointed out that the nervous system is never at rest, and the patterns of neural activation constantly change. When sensory information reaches the spinal cord it enters a system that is already active. The existing activity influences the fate of incoming sensory information, sometimes amplifying it and sometimes decreasing the incoming neural signals. These complex modulations in the spinal cord and brain can affect the perception of pain. Although the theory was later extended by Melzack (1992) to place stronger emphasis on the role of the brain in pain perception (neuromatrix theory), the influence of experience and expectation in the perception of pain have become central to our understanding of the pain experience. The physiology of pain is covered elsewhere in this book (*Chapter 2*), but the key point here is the move towards a biopsychosocial model of pain. The gate control theory explains the influence of cognitive aspects of pain, by hypothesising central control mechanisms that affect sensory input, as well as being affected by it. If the emotional status of the person is negative (eg. anxious, worried, depressed), this can increase pain by affecting the central control trigger and, thus, open the gate; while positive emotional states brought about by distraction and relaxation cause the gate to close, and so reduce the sensation of pain.

These theoretical debates on the meaning of pain are not merely an academic exercise, as this new understanding of pain has led to calls for changes in treatment, and created pressure to treat pain as a symptom or disorder in its own right. In 1979, the sub-committee for taxonomy of the International Association for the Study of Pain (IASP) drafted a definition of pain as, 'an unpleasant sensory and emotional experience associated with actual or potential tissue damage, or described in terms of such damage' (p. 250). This definition clearly covers both the physical and emotional components of the pain experience, and reflects the currently held belief that personal perception mediates the experience of pain.

Psychological factors in pain perception

There has been a growing recognition that pain is a complex perceptual experience influenced by a wide range of psychosocial factors, including emotions, sociocultural background, the meaning of pain to that person, beliefs, attitudes, and expectations. For some people, pain can be an everyday experience which becomes a useful sign of damage, prompting individuals to act.

Pain that persists for months will influence all aspects of a person's functioning as it interferes with planned behaviour. For those in chronic pain, the extent of damage does not necessarily relate to the pain experience. Some people report pain that has no identifiable source, while others with clear tissue damage do not report pain (Eccleston, 2001). Given that pain can be experienced distal to the site of damage, or in a missing limb, it is clear that pain is not a reliable indicator of tissue damage, nor is tissue damage a reliable indicator of pain. We know that people are different and will respond to pain differently — as well as differing in their attempts to manage it. Trying to understand what predicts these differences can lead to improvements in the way we deliver treatment, as well as improve the effectiveness of interventions.

Early research into the psychology of pain concentrated on global issues, such as personality, age, gender, and cultural differences. However, research reviewed by Eccleston (2001), indicates that the evidence of these broad-sweeping characteristics is limited and inconclusive. More recent research, discussed below, has focused on more specific aspects of personality, and these studies have been more enlightening.

Patient beliefs

There is growing evidence that patients' beliefs affect their perception of pain (Turk and Okifuji, 2002). Beliefs about what symptoms mean, the individual's ability to control their pain, and concern about the future can all influence pain perception and response to treatment (Tota-Faucette et al, 1993; Schmidl, 2000). In many elderly patients, there is a belief that pain comes with age and must be expected, leading to an acceptance of high levels of pain being normal.

When we first injure ourselves, resting and protecting the area is appropriate adaptive behaviour. However, relying on this approach in a chronic pain situation is often maladaptive, as it can result in a fear of taking exercise which has a rehabilitative function. Responding to chronic pain in this way can also lead to a preoccupation with bodily symptoms, and a focus on somatic experiences that might otherwise be ignored. This results in the person avoiding more and more activity in the belief that it will perpetuate further problems.

The cause of the pain can influence both patients and healthcare professionals. Patients who experience pain following an accident tend to view physical sensation as harmful (thus increasing their anxiety); while patients who report symptoms following trauma are five times more likely to be prescribed opioid medication than those with an accidental injury as the cause, even when there is no difference in physical damage (Turk and Okifuji, 1996). This suggests that the beliefs of both patients and healthcare professionals can influence pain management options.

Fear

People are fearful of pain, so it is natural to avoid fear-provoking events. For example, if you find injections painful you will explore every other option of drug delivery! However, where the threat of pain is constant (eg. a person experiencing pain every time they move), a pattern of vigilance to pain can develop. McCracken (1997) found that patients who pay a lot of attention to pain, also report higher pain intensity, increased use of health resources, and more emotional distress. Excessive attention may explain poor concentration observed in patients with fibromyalgia (Rollman and Lautenbacher, 1993). As Waddell *et al* (1993) argue, the fear of pain is more disabling than pain itself. Accounts of being in chronic pain reveal a fear of a life overtaken by pain (Carr *et al*, 2005).

Worry/anxiety

Worrying about pain, its causes and consequences, is a common experience for those in chronic pain (de Vlieger *et al*, 2006). Aldrich *et al* (2000) have investigated the concept of 'worry' in terms of its function, and have focused on the way in which patients focus attention on pain as a central 'problem' that has to be solved. The difficulty for such patients is that pain may not have a readily accessible, easy solution; hence, worrying can become intense and uncontrollable. This 'chronic worrying' can have a negative effect on an individual's ability to problem solve — and consequently, individuals can lose their confidence in their ability to problem solve. Recent research (de Vlieger *et al*, 2006) involving 185 adults with chronic pain (63 of whom were consecutively recruited from a tertiary chronic pain centre, while the others were responders to advertisements for those in pain, but not under the care of a healthcare professional), investigated 'worrying' and related problem-solving, and found no differences between those attending a specialist clinic and non-patients. However, the study also showed that worrying was significantly related to depression, catastrophic thoughts about pain, and disability.

'Catastrophic thinking' is a response to threatening pain, which seems to predict the intensity of pain, and is associated with more pronounced pain behaviour, heightened emotional distress and greater disability (Sullivan *et al*, 2001; Keefe *et al*, 2004). Basically, 'catastrophic thinking' means an almost immediate appraisal of a situation as extremely or globally catastrophic, such that the person magnifies the outcome and the effects of pain, while minimising their ability to cope. Aldrich *et al* (2000) have proposed that this is an extreme form of normal worry about pain. They also report a cyclic relationship in these situations, as chronic worry/anxiety about pain and how to solve the problem of pain may, in turn, lead to a pattern of catastrophic thinking.

Catastrophic thinking is associated with increased attention to the source of the pain. Crombez *et al* (1998) have demonstrated that those with catastrophic thoughts were unable to distract themselves from a threatening painful stimulus. This finding was confirmed by Van Damme *et al* (2004) in a human volunteer study of 37 undergraduates, who concluded that high pain catastrophisers had great difficulty in disengaging from pain. This may have important implications for therapy — given that distraction is a technique that is often used as a positive way of coping with pain. Those with catastrophic thoughts about pain may not respond at all to this type of intervention, which suggests that distraction techniques, either alone or as part of a cognitive behavioural package, should not be used with this group (Goubert *et al*, 2004).

Catastrophic thinking is considered to be a multidimensional concept involving three key concepts: rumination, magnification and helplessness (Osman *et al*, 2000; Sullivan *et al*, 2000). To date, there is limited research to indicate which of these three elements relates most closely to the experience of pain. Sullivan *et al* (2005) have shown that catastrophic thinking is a significant factor of the pain experience

(80 patients with neuropathic pain were included in this study, 19 of whom had diabetic neuropathy), and that helplessness was the strongest predictor of spontaneous pain (as measured by the McGill Pain Questionnaire, Melzack, 1987). They explain their findings in terms of living with a condition with relatively ineffective treatments, which leads to a helpless orientation towards pain and an inability to cope. Alternatively, living with someone who continually expresses helplessness in the face of their condition can be difficult, and this may lead to a breakdown in interpersonal relationships and the positive support that others can provide (Cano *et al*, 2004).

Living with chronic pain is a perfect situation in which worry can develop and grow, and is a common feature of the chronic pain experience. Those who worry about their pain are not passive in this experience, but constantly ruminate on the endless possible consequences of potentially painful threats, and look for multiple solutions to living with pain — some will catastrophise about future pain experiences and their ability to cope. The difficulty for healthcare professionals is that many of these problems may be difficult to solve, and yet progress will only be made via active involvement, usually through cognitive behavioural therapy (CBT).

Mood state

Those who live with others in chronic, persistent pain would not be surprised to learn that the majority of patients who present at a pain clinic, also present with some degree of depression. However, this depression is not directly related to the pain, but to the disabling consequences of how the individual reacts to pain (Turk *et al*, 1995). Two important aspects of depression relevant to this patient group are anger and self-denigration.

❖ *Anger* is not always part of depression, but some chronic pain patients are extremely angry. The anger is difficult to express as there is no clear or immediate target for the anger, but it is related to global feelings of frustration and of 'being blamed'. Anger can have a negative effect on treatment, as aggression and hostility are difficult to deal with and often result in the patient, or the healthcare professional, withdrawing from the therapy sessions (which, in turn, leads to more anger). Some authors (eg. Wade *et al*, 1990) have called for the explicit treatment of anger to be included in a range of other interventions.

❖ *Self-denigration* refers to the negative thoughts that those with depression express about their self-worth (eg. 'I'll never be able to control this pain'). Although research in this area is relatively new, there are important lessons for treatment from this information. Simply suggesting to patients that the route to successful management lies in themselves, may be an invitation to fail — as depressed individuals already feel useless and pathetic. However, dealing with the depression and the associated thought patterns, may help to increase the success of treatment of pain.

Coping with pain

Many patients who present with chronic pain often present with a range of other problems, including sleep disruption and fatigue (Moldofsky and Lue, 1993). Sleep and pain have a bi-directional relationship; pain interferes with sleep, but tiredness increases our awareness of pain. Many of these patients become isolated, with unsatisfactory roles within their families. Chronic, persistent pain, fear and depression lead to a negative impact on other types of thinking, including poor concentration, poor memory, and failure to complete cognitive tasks (Dufton, 1989). When faced with this ongoing stressful situation, individuals attempt to cope in a number of ways.

The issue of taking control has received a great deal of attention, and research has shown that when patients are given control over their own pain medication, it can lead to reduced pain, reduced tiredness, and increased energy. This can be seen even when the control is only over the monitoring of pain, and not active medication control (Leventhal *et al*, 1989). Some patients prefer not to think about forthcoming painful events, but try to think of something else; while others focus on predicting the effects of pain in order to deal with them. Eccleston (2001) concludes that both approaches can work, but only those strategies that fit with the person's preference for dealing with the situation will be effective.

Most people living with chronic pain struggle to make sense of the experience. Coping with such a situation is only effective once the individual has understood the experience within their own system of knowledge (ie. the way in which they understand the world and how it works). People need to 'get their head around' the fact that they may have to live in pain. Those who are most resistant to psychological support are those patients who repeatedly present for help with their pain, but have no known aetiology. The 'not knowing' leads to more distress, and without a diagnosis we develop an increased belief that the pain represents severe illness (Cioffi, 1991).

The experience of pain is complex and multifactorial. Individuals respond to chronic pain in a number of ways, both in terms of how they appraise the situation and how they cope. The move towards a biopsychosocial model of understanding pain should help healthcare professionals deal with the emotional component of pain, as well as focusing on the treatment of the sensory perception of pain.

Pain in patients with chronic wounds

There is increasing evidence that patients with a range of chronic wounds experience high levels of constant, persistent pain, as well as pain from the interventions necessary to care for their wounds (eg. dressing changes). Persoon *et al* (2004), in a systematic review of the impact of living with leg ulcers, reviewed 37 papers and concluded that leg ulcers pose a major threat to physical functioning. Although pain is not the only symptom of the wound that the patients have to deal with, there is little doubt that pain has a major impact on everyday living.

If we put this finding in context, healthcare professionals need to be aware that this group of predominantly frail, elderly patients, face major psychological adaptation (Price, 2006), as they have to cope with a range of issues related to symptom management (Flanagan *et al*, 2006; Hopkins 2004; Neil and Munjas, 2000), and deal with fragmented service provision (Husband, 2001).

Not only is there evidence that patients report pain when they are asked about their everyday lives, but some studies have provided evidence of the scale of the problem. In 1997, Hofman *et al* investigated 140 consecutive patients at two centres (Oxford and Uppsala, Sweden), and found that 64% of patients with venous leg ulcers reported severe pain and, in 38% of those patients, the pain was continuous. This is a startling figure, particularly in a group that have traditionally been thought not to experience pain; indeed, years ago, lack of pain was part of the differential diagnosis for venous ulceration. These figures have been confirmed by other researchers in other countries: Noonan and Burge (1998) report that 88% of their sample of 51 reported intermittent pain, and for 12% it was continuous; Wissing *et al* (2002) report that 63% of their 70 cases had ulcer-related pain; and a Canadian study with a sample of 255, report a point prevalence of around 50% (Nemeth *et al*, 2003). In these studies, around 50% of those who reported pain were treated pharmacologically, with between 10 and 50% of patients using morphine-based analgesia.

Although there is more evidence on the importance of pain to patients with leg ulcers than those with other chronic wound types, there is some evidence that pain is also a problem for those with pressure ulceration. Quirino *et al* (2003) report on a qualitative study from America in 20 patients with Grade I–II (National Pressure Ulcer Advisory Panel [NPUAP]) pressure ulcers at the sacrum. All the patients reported pain and 80% reported that it was continuous. Seventy-four percent of those treated pharmacologically reported that the treatment had little or no effect.

The concern of healthcare professionals about the extent of this problem is demonstrated in two documents. In 2002, the European Wound Management Association (EWMA) produced a position document on pain, outlining some of the important principles for the understanding of pain, and also outlining some treatment options. In 2004, the World Union of Wound Healing Societies (WUWHS) produced a consensus statement on key issues related to minimising pain at dressing change. Both these documents represent an important step forward in our understanding of pain as applied to this patient group. Unfortunately, the psychological aspects of pain, its perception and treatment in this group of patients have yet to be fully investigated. However, there are lessons that can be learnt from the chronic pain world that show that a few changes to clinical practice can have a beneficial impact on patients.

Psychological approaches to pain management

In many acute pain situations, pain management is dictated by the attending clinician, and the role of psychological approaches is limited. However, when dealing with those in chronic, persistent pain, psychological factors cannot be avoided and are of vital importance. This is especially so for those who have lived with chronic, persistent pain for many months, as they will be distressed and will probably have already tried a range of treatment options.

Table 9.1 outlines a range of ways in which knowledge of the psychological factors associated with the pain experience can be used by the clinician to maximise the benefits of assessment and treatment. Relatively small changes in how information is requested and care is delivered can have a profound impact on the patient.

There are also a number of ways in which psychological support can be provided to patients, to complement the more traditional pharmacological approaches. Patients often reject, and carers are sometimes reluctant to accept, pharmacological interventions for pain on the basis of fear of addiction; concern about side-effects; a belief that pain signifies disease progression; or a belief that they should not complain about pain. Alternatively, some patients prefer to deal with the psychosocial aspects of care on a personal basis and reject the interventions of healthcare professionals, despite an empathic response to their situation. Yet research has demonstrated that psychological factors play an important role in patients' coping abilities, how they maintain their quality of life, and their resultant disability from chronic pain (Schmidl, 2000; Turk and Okifuji, 2002).

The form of psychological intervention with the most evidence related to success is cognitive behavioural therapy. This is a term used to describe a programme of therapy that is a collaboration between the therapist and patient to work on how people think and behave in relation to pain. Much of the treatment is based on the 'here-and-now', and there is an assumption that the main goal of the therapy is to help patients bring about desired changes in their lives. The first principle of cognitive behavioural assessment is that an individual's behaviour is determined by their immediate situation, and their interpretation of that situation (for example, many patients see pain as dominating their lives and find it difficult to see how this can change without pharmacological intervention). The programme is always time-limited, with clearly agreed goals. A programme should include positive reinforcement of 'well' behaviour, increasing general fitness, and develop insight into the nature of self-defeating thought patterns and the 'evidence' that individuals use to justify them.

Table 9.1: Psychological factors in clinical use

Psychological factor	Implications for patient	Implications for practice
Avoidance	Patients will try to avoid pain and painful procedures. A pattern of avoidance may emerge, which can lead to chronic pain	Be aware of this, and plan for it. Try to explain that pain does not necessarily mean 'damage' or 'disease'; this message must be given by someone who has credibility for the patient
Awareness of the pain	Patients will have impaired concentration and possibly poor memory – their train of thought is constantly interrupted by pain. Patients may talk about the pain frequently	Keep messages clear and brief. Build in opportunities to repeat messages. Be consistent with messages. Do not assume that if a patient talks about their pain a lot, that they are showing signs of hypochondria
Mood state	The patient may be depressed or angry. They may shout at carers or retreat into themselves. This group is particularly likely to have broken concentration.	Be patient – depression and anger often push others away. Make sure that all options for the depression have been covered, including pharmacological support. This group are less likely to have received help and information; those who are angry are likely to be particularly confused
Making sense of pain	In terms of pain, what makes sense to one person may not help another. Patients struggle to understand the causes of pain, and those without a diagnosis will fear disease and illness	Ask patients about their understanding of the causes of their pain and its time-course. Be aware that their understanding of their pain will influence their behaviour. Try to give meaningful information about the duration of treatment and a possible time-course for the pain
Involve the patient	One way of coping successfully with pain is to take some control over the process — this may be through distraction or information gathering	Match your interventions to the usual way the patient deals with pain — if they seek information, provide information on what they should expect and how long the pain will last (always overestimate)

Adapted from Eccleston, 2001

There have been several systematic reviews of cognitive behavioural therapy for adults with chronic pain (Flor *et al*, 1992; Turner *et al*, 1996; Malone and Strube, 1988, Morley *et al*, 1999; Eccleston, 2001), each of which concluded that there is good evidence of effectiveness, especially when compared with no-treatment controls or education alone. However, there is also evidence that the success of cognitive behavioural therapy is dependent on the experience and quality of the therapist. In a time of scant resources for the health service, it is unlikely that recent calls for the routine inclusion of cognitive behavioural therapy in pain clinics will be met (Audit Commission, 1998), particularly given the lack of appropriately qualified staff.

Healthcare professionals should encourage patients to become involved in coping skills training, behavioural contracts, biofeedback, relaxation and distraction techniques, or social support/self-help groups. Help in organising their day to include exercise, socialisation, TV, music and relaxation, can encourage patients to take more control and improve their coping ability. Although there has been little specific research on psychological interventions for pain in wound care, a recent trial of a community intervention programme showed pain level improvements and improved ulcer healing where there was extra focus on information sharing and preventive care for the patient (Edwards *et al*, 2005). This approach could be a model to help with the considerable emotional aspects of wound pain.

Conclusion

Pain stems from both physiological and psychological factors. The degree of tissue damage may contribute to a person's experience of pain, but personal perceptions are frequently more important. Acute pain is often adaptive and there is a limited, although important role for psychology in this process. However, in chronic, persistent pain situations, the pain may continue beyond the point of healing and is often experienced in the absence of detectable tissue damage, and psychological interventions may be of real benefit. For the patient with wound pain, simple changes in clinical practice, based on an awareness of the important psychological factors that may influence the pain experience, can result in major improvements for the patient. Healthcare professionals must be aware that the wound pain experience will not only relate to the acute pain experienced during treatment interventions (eg. dressing change, debridement), but may also exist as chronic, persistent pain which dominates the lives of their patients. Awareness of the benefits of psychological interventions, especially as part of a package of pain-related care, may lead to major improvements in the everyday lives of those living with chronic wounds.

References

Aldrich S, Eccleston C, Crombez G (2000) Worrying about chronic pain: vigilance to threat and misdirected problem solving. *Behav Res Ther* **38**: 457–70

Audit Commission (1998) *Anaesthetic Services in the UK*. Department of Health, London

Beecher HK (1946) Pain of men wounded in battle. *Ann Surg* **123**: 96–105

Beecher HK (1956) Relationship of significance of wound to pain experienced. *J Am Med Assoc* **161**(17): 1609–13

Brannon L, Feist J (1997) *Health Psychology: An introduction to behaviour and health*. Brooks/Cole Publishing Company, Pacific Grove

Cano A, Gillis M, Heinz W, Geisser M, Foran H (2004) Marital functioning, chronic pain, and psychological distress. *Pain* **107**: 99–106

Carr D, Loeser JJ, Thomas DK (2005) *Narrative, Pain and Suffering*. IASP Press, Seattle, WA

Cioffi D (1991) Asymmetry of doubt in medical self-diagnosis: the ambiguity of 'uncertain wellness'. *J Pers Soc Psychol* **61**: 969–80

Crombez G, Eccleston C, Baeyens F, Eelen P (1998) When somatic information threatens, catastrophic thinking enhances attentional interference. *Pain* **75**: 187–98

De Vlieger P, Crombez G, Eccleston C (2006) Worrying about chronic pain: an examination of worry and problem-solving in adults who identify as chronic pain sufferers. *Pain* **120**: 138–44

Dufton BD (1989) Cognitive failure and chronic pain. *Int J Psychiatry Med* **19**: 291–7

Eccleston C (2001) Role of psychology in pain management. *Br J Anaesthesia* **87**(1): 144–52

Edwards H, Courtney M, Findlayson K, Lindsay E, Lewis C, Shuter P, Chang A (2005) Chronic venous leg ulcers: Effect of a community nursing intervention on pain and healing. *Nurs Standard* **19**: 47–54

European Wound Management Association (EWMA) (2002) *Position Document: Pain at wound dressing changes*. Medical Education Partnership Ltd, Londonn

Flanagan M, Vogensen H, Haase L (2006) Case series investigating the experience of pain in patients with chronic venous leg ulcers treated with a foam dressing releasing ibuprofen. *Wound Wide Wounds*

Flor H, Fydrich T, Turk DC (1992) Efficacy of multidisciplinary pain treatment centers: a meta-analytic review. *Pain* **49**: 221–30

Goubert L, Crombez G, Eccleston C, Devaulder J (2004) Distration from chronic pain during a pain-inducing activity is associated with greater post-activity pain. *Pain* 110: 220–7

Hofman D, Arnold F, Cherry G, Lindholm S, Glynn C (1997) Pain in venous leg ulcers. *J Wound Care* 6(5): 222–4

Hopkins A (2004) Disrupted lives: investigating coping strategies for non-healing leg ulcers. *Br J Nurs* 13(9): 556–63

Husband LL (2001) Shaping the trajectory of patients with venous ulceration in primary care. *Health Expectations* 4(3): 189–98

International Association for the Study of Pain (IASP), subcommittee on Taxonomy (1979) Pain terms: A list with definitions and notes on usage. *Pain* 6: 249–52

Keefe FJ, Rumble ME, Scipio CD, Giordano LA, Perri LM (2004) Psychological aspects of persistent pain: current state of the science. *J Pain* 5(4): 195–211

Leventhal EA, Leventhal H, Shacham S, Easterling DV (1989) Active coping reduces reports of pain from childbirth. *J Consul Clin Psychol* 57: 365–71

McCracken LM (1997) Attention to pain in persons with chronic pain: a behavioural approach. *Behav Ther* 28: 271–84

Malone MD, Strube MJ (1988) Meta-analysis of non-medical treatments for chronic pain. *Pain* 34: 231–44

Melzack R (1987) The short-form McGill pain questionnaire. *Pain* 30: 191–7

Melzack MD (1992) Phantom limbs. *Sci Am* 266(4): 120–6

Melzack R, Wall PD (1965) Pain mechanisms: a new theory. *Science* 150: 971–9

Melzack R, Wall PD, Ty TC (1982) Acute pain in an emergency clinic: latency of onset and descriptor patterns. *Pain* 14: 33–43

Melzack R, Wall PD (1988) *The Challenge of Pain*. Penguin, London

Moldofsky H, Lue F (1993) Disordered sleep, pain, fatigue and gastrointestinal symptoms in fibromyalgia: chronic fatigue and irritable bowel syndromes. In Mayer EA, Raybould HE, eds. *Basic and Clinical Aspects of Chronic Abdominal Pain*. Elsevier Science Publishers, New York: 249–55

Morley S, Eccleston C, Williams A (1999) Systematic review and meta-analysis of randomised controlled trials of cognitive behaviour therapy and behaviour therapy for chronic pain in adults, excluding headache. *Pain* 80: 1–13

Neil JA, Munjas BA (2000) Living with a chronic wound: The voices of sufferers. *Ostomy/Wound Management* 46(5):28–38

Nemeth KA, Harrison MB, Graham ID, Burke S (2003) Pain in pure and mixed aetiology venous leg ulcers: a three phase point prevalence study. *J Wound Care* 12(9): 336–40

Noonan L, Burge S (1998) Venous leg ulcers: is pain a problem? *Phlebology* 13: 14–19

Osman A, Barrois FX, Kopper BA, Hauptmann W, Jones J, O'Neill E (2000) The pain catastrophizing scale; further psychometric evaluation with an adult sample. *J Behav Med* 23: 351–65

Persoon A, Heinen MM, van der Vleuten CJ, de Rooij MJ, van de Kerkhof PC, van Achterberg T (2004) Leg ulcers: a review of their impact on daily life. *J Clin Nurs* 13(3): 341–54

Price P (2006) Psychosocial issues related to chronic wounds. In: Morrison M, Moffat C, Franks P, eds. *Leg Ulcers: A problem-based learning approach.* Elsevier Science Publishers, New York

Quirino J, Santo V, Quednau T, Martins A, Lima P, Almeida M (2003) Pain in pressure ulcers. *Wounds* 15(12): 381–9

Rollmann GB, Lautenbacher S (1993) Hypervigilance effects in fibromylagia: pain experience and pain perception. In: Voeroy H, Merskey H, eds. *Progress in Fibromyalgia and Mysfascial Pain.* Elsevier Science Publishers, New York: 149–59

Schmidl F (2000) Psychological concepts and treatments for chronic pain and somatoform syndromes. *Wien Med Wochenschr* 150: 295–9

Sullivan MJL, Tripp D, Rogers W, Spanish W (2000) Catastrophizing and pain perception in sports participants. *J Applied Sport Psychology* 12: 151–67

Sullivan MJL, Thorn B, Haythornthwaite JA, Keefe FJ, Martin M, Bradley LA (2001) Theoretical perspectives on the relation between catastrophizing and pain. *Clin J Pain* 17: 52–64

Sullivan MJL, Lynch ME, Clark AJ (2005) Dimensions of catastrophic thinking associated with pain experience and disability in patients with neuropathic pain conditions. *Pain* 113: 310–15

Tota-Faucette ME, Gil KM, Williams DA, Keefe FJ, Goli V (1993) Predictors of response to pain management treatment; the role of family environment and changes in cognitive processes. *Clin J Pain* 9: 115–23

Turk DC, Okifuji A, Scharff L (1995) Chronic pain and depression — role of perceived impact and perceived control in different age cohorts. *Pain* 61: 93–101

Turk DC, Okifuji A (1996) Perception of traumatic onset, compensation status and physical findings; impact on severity of pain, emotional distress and disability in chronic pain patients. *J Behav Med* 19: 435

Turk DC, Okifuji A (2002) Psychological factors in chronic pain: evolution and revolution. *J Consult Clin Psychol* **70**(3): 678–90

Turner JA, Schroth WS, Fordyce WE (1996) Educational and behavioural interventions for back pain in primary care. *Spine* **21**: 2851–9

Van Damme S, Crombez G, Eccleston C (2004) Disengagement from pain: the role of catastrophic thinking about pain. *Pain* **107**: 70–6

Waddell G, Newton M, Henderson I, Somerville D, Main CJ (1993) A fear-avoidance beliefs questionnaire (FABQ) and the role of fear-avoidance beliefs in chronic low-back-pain and disability. *Pain* **52**: 157–68

Wade JB, Price DD, Hamer RM, Schwartz SM, Hart RP (1990) An emotional component analysis of chronic pain. *Pain* **40**: 303–10

Wissing U, Ek AC, Unosson M (2002) Life situation and function in elderly people with and without leg ulcers. *Scand J Caring Sciences* **16**(1): 59–65

World Union of Wound Healing Societies (2004) *Principles of Best Practice: Minimising pain at wound dressing-related procedures. A consensus document.* Available online at: www.wuwhs.org/pdf/consensus_eng.pdf

CHAPTER 10

AN EXPLORATION OF RECENT GUIDELINES AND DOCUMENTS TO GUIDE PRACTICE

David Gray, Pam Cooper and Keith Harding

Wound pain is an issue that distresses patients, and has appeared in the literature relating to wound management for a number of years. The issue is not confined to any particular aetiology or type of wound. The work of Krasner (1996), Hoffman *et al* (1997), Rook (1998), Noonan and Burge (1998), all established that wounds were potentially painful, and that wound pain was largely unaddressed in many patients.

The past few years has seen the publication of statements and guidelines that relate to the management of pain in wound management. Initially, the focus was on pain at dressing changes alone, but recent publications have broadened the debate to include the issue of pain in wounds for the patient. *Table 10.1* lists the publications that are examined further in this chapter.

The plethora of guidelines seen in the past four years are indicative of the problem and show that practitioners, researchers, patients and industry are working to provide solutions to manage pain and suffering for patients.

This chapter examines the major documents related to wound pain, highlighting the key points in each document, and indicating the common, or red thread, that runs through each of the documents.

Table 10.1: Wound pain publications

Year	Title of document	Type of document
2002	Pain at wound dressing changes	European Wound Management Association (EWMA), Position Document
2003	Practical treatment of wound pain and trauma: a patient-centred approach	Continuing medical education document
2004	Minimising pain at wound dressing-related procedures. A consensus document	World Union of Wound Healing Societies (WUWHS) Consensus Document. Principles of Best Practice
2004	Issues in Paediatric Wound Care. Minimising trauma and pain	Multidisciplinary advisory group report. Sponsored by an educational grant from the Tendra Academy, Mölnlycke Health Care
2004	Independent Advisory Group. Best Practice Statement Minimising Trauma and Pain in Wound Management. Wounds UK Ltd, 2004. Available online at: www.wounds-uk.com	Report of an independent advisory group developed by specialists within the field of tissue viability within the UK. Sponsored by an educational grant from the Tendra Academy, Mölnlycke Health Care and endorsed by the Tissue Viability Nurses Association
2005	Issues in Neonatal Wound Care. Minimising Trauma and Pain	Independent advisory group report. Sponsored by an educational grant from the Tendra Academy, Mölnlycke Health Care
2005	Pain at wound dressing-related procedures: a template for assessment	Clinical paper
2006	Issues in Wound Care: Implementing Best Practice to Minimise Trauma and Pain	Report from a Tendra Academy Expert Form. Sponsored by an educational grant from the Tendra Academy, Mölnlycke Health Care

The first major document was the European Wound Management Association (EWMA) Position Paper published in 2002. This document marked a major step forward in the recognition of pain in wound management as, for the first time, a major wound association established a clear position on the assessment, management and treatment of wound-related pain. The introduction indicated the EWMA view that the association wished to provide clear advice on the clinical management of a specific area of wound care. The concentration on pain at dressing change is understandable. Moffatt *et al* (2002), in a survey on wound pain, showed that pain at dressing change was an area that practitioners in this multinational study rated as the time of greatest pain. The document has three major sections. Section 1 uses this study (2002) to present an overview of wound pain and the size of the problem. Section 2 examines and explains the theories behind pain. The role of the nervous system in relation to tissue damage is also explained, alongside the psychosocial aspects relating to pain perception and awareness in individuals. The importance of the gate control theory is explained in the linking of the physical and psychological elements of pain. Section 3 is a guide to management, the major points are summarised in *Table 10.2*.

In 2003, the 'Practical treatment of wound pain and trauma: a patient-centered approach' was published in *Ostomy/Wound Management* (OWM) (Reddy *et al*, 2003). The piece was primarily a continuing medical education document for North American practitioners, but it built significantly on the EWMA document (2002). Separate sections give an overview of wound pain, followed by sections on pain in leg ulcers, diabetic foot ulcers, and pressure ulcers. The document uses the EWMA Position Paper as a framework, adding case studies from a North American perspective. The document has been superseded by a newer supplement, 'When Wound Care Hurts: The Importance of Addressing the Pain' (*Ostomy/Wound Management* 51(11A) suppl, 2005).

2004 saw the publication of a number of documents, including the World Union of Wound Healing Societies (WUWHS) consensus document, 'Minimising pain at wound dressing-related procedures'. The introduction to this document recognises the significance of the previous two documents and comments on the size and significance of the problem, alongside clear statements on the implications for practice. Of the documents listed, this one is by far the most comprehensive and far reaching. The use of this document could influence the change of practice in local situations. A review is presented in *Table 10.3*.

Table 10.2: EWMA Position paper, section 3

Section	Sub-section	Key points	Guides for practice
Scale of the problem		Several studies show that dressing change may exacerbate pain	Effective pain management strategies should be considered for all patients indicating wound pain
Pain models		Krasner (1995) presents a model that indicates that pain can be caused by treatment, but also a background pain element exists	Practitioners should not just consider procedural pain, but should also make themselves aware of the affective and cognitive components of pain
	Dimensions of pain	Sensory component	The physical stimulus of pain
		Affective component	Any negative feelings associated with pain that may affect the patient's current perception, ie. feeling depressed or irritable, lacking sleep. These are all things that may exacerbate negative pain feelings
		Cognitive dimension	The attitudes and beliefs that may influence a person's feelings of pain and their coping mechanisms, ie. previous painful dressing changes
		Socio-cultural dimension	The impact of long-standing pain on the networks, beliefs, and cultural or religious factors may also have an influence
Pain assessment		There is no magic solution for all situations	
	Existing wound pain	Assessment of pain should include questioning and observation of response. A recognised pain intensity scale should be used to establish the severity of the pain. Whatever scale is used, or chosen locally, its use should be consistent if the patient indicates they are in pain	Pain assessment, including intensity and severity, should form part of a baseline assessment for all individuals with a wound. Use of an agreed pain rating scale should be part of local practice. Some form of active intervention to reduce pain should be taken to reduce pain before procedures take place
	Neuropathic pain	Management of this kind of pain often involves a specialist referral	Be aware of local care pathways for such patients

Table 10.2: EWMA Position paper, section 3 cont.

Section	Sub-section	Key points	Guides for practice
	Socio-cultural issues/ anxiety	The history of the patient's pain is important in shaping their experience	Establish what the patient believes is the cause of the pain and what relieves it
	Analgesia	Analgesia alone will only reduce intensity, and for a limited time	Use a combination of strategies to reduce pain intensity Analgesic use should follow the WHO analgesic ladder. Step1: NSAID or local topical treatment Step 2: Add a mild opioid (use oral medication if possible) Step 3: replace mild opioid with potent opioid
	Reducing anxiety	Anxiety is reduced in the same way as pain	The reduction of anxiety
	Dressing selection and removal	Dressing selection should use products that minimise pain at dressing change. The prevailing wound conditions should not be ignored	Strategies for the relief of pain at dressing change: 1. Avoid any unnecessary stimulus to the wound 2. Handle wounds gently, be aware that any small touch can cause pain 3. Select a dressing which: a. is appropriate for the type of wound b. maintains moist wound healing c. minimises pain and trauma on removal d. remains *in situ* long enough to reduce change frequency 4. Reconsider your choice if: a. trauma or pain or bleeding are experienced on removal b. soaking is required to remove the product
	Ongoing assessment	Pain reassessment should be a normal part of the treatment cycle	The condition of a wound may change, as may the patient's pain intensity and perception. The effectiveness of any intervention should be monitored and adjusted at every reassessment if necessary

Table 10.3: WUWHS Consensus Document: Minimising pain at wound dressing-related procedures

Section	Sub-section	Key points	Guides for practice
Principles of Best Practice	Understanding types of pain	Nociceptive and neuropathic pain	APPLICATION TO PRACTICE Assume all wounds are painful Over time wounds may become more painful Accept that the skin surrounding the wound can become sensitive and painful Accept that for some patients the lightest touch, or simply air moving across the wound can be intensely painful Know when to refer for specialist assessment
Causes of pain			*Psychosocial factors:* eg. age, gender, culture, education, mental state – anxiety, depression, fear, loss/grief *Environmental factors:* eg. timing of procedure, setting – level of noise/positioning of patient, resources *Operative:* cutting of tissue or prolonged manipulation normally requiring anaesthetic, eg. debridement, major burn dressings *Procedural:* routine/basic interventions, eg. dressing removal, wound cleansing, dressing application *Incident:* movement-related activities, eg. friction, dressing slippage, coughing *Background:* persistent underlying pain due to wound aetiology, local wound factors, eg. ischaemia, infection
Assessment of pain	Initial assessment	Should be carried out by an experienced practitioner, and should obtain a comprehensive history	Ensure that each pain assessment is individualised, relevant and does not become an additional stressor
	Ongoing assessment	Should be carried out at each dressing change	Pain should be assessed before and after any interventions or dressing changes
	Review assessment	Should be carried out by an experienced practitioner	Forms part of a major reassessment or case review. Factors that influence pain both positively and negatively should be documented. Pain scoring over time may help reveal trends that can influence treatment decisions
Assessment strategies	Pain is what the patient says it is	Sometimes the patient does not say	Assessment strategies should include observation and an understanding of common pain descriptors. Some questions to assist in the assessment of pain are in Box 10.1

Table 10.3 : WUWHS Consensus Document: Minimising pain at wound dressing-related procedures cont.

Section	Sub-section	Key points	Guides for practice
	Measuring pain	Pain should be graded, not just a simple do you have pain or not	Pain scores should be used routinely in assessment. A pain score of less than 4 should be a target. Scores that persist above 4 should prompt a change in pain management. Pain diaries may prove useful for some patients in determining an overall pain profile. Assume all patients can use a rating scale until proven otherwise, routine pain scoring during dressing-related procedures can significantly impact on management. A selection of pain assessment tools is shown in Wong et al, 2001
	Professional issues	Patients have a right to expect a minimum standard of care and treatment	Issues of accountability need to be explored by practitioners treating painful wounds. If a treatment or procedure is painful, it is negligent to repeat it. Remember that a patient's previous experience of pain can determine their expression of pain at a later date
Management of pain	Treat underlying cause	Treat the patient as a whole, not just the wound	
		Address local wound factors that may also cause pain	**Local wound factors:** These include ischaemia, infection, excessive dryness or excessive exudate, oedema, dermatological problems, and maceration of the surrounding skin
		Consider analgesic options	The WHO analgesic pain ladder STEP 1: Non-Opioid ± adjuvant STEP 2: Opioid for mild to moderate pain (± non-Opioid/adjuvant) STEP 3: Opioid for moderate to severe pain (± non-Opioid/adjuvant) Note: Depending on the pain assessment, it may be appropriate to start at a higher step
		Key management points	Background pain and incident pain must be well controlled to minimise pain intensity at wound dressing-related procedures effectively. The clinician must act early to relieve pain and prevent provoking pain. If an intervention, such as dressing removal or wound cleansing is causing increasing pain requiring more aggressive analgesia, the clinician must reconsider treatment choices

Table 10.3 :WUWHS Consensus Document: Minimising pain at wound dressing-related procedures cont.		
Section	**Sub-section**	**Key points**
		Guides for practice
	Procedural pain	

Procedural interventions

There is a vast array of dressing-related procedures. Specific interventions will require specific management, but the following general principles should be considered:

● Be aware of current status of pain
● Know and avoid, where possible, pain triggers
● Know and use, where possible, pain reducers
● Avoid unnecessary manipulation of the wound
● Explore simple patient-controlled techniques, such as counting up and down, focusing on the breath entering and leaving the lungs or listening to music
● Reconsider management choices if pain becomes intolerable and document as an adverse event
● Observe the wound and the surrounding skin for evidence of infection, necrosis, maceration, etc
● Consider the temperature of the product or solution before applying to the wound
● Avoid excessive pressure from a dressing, bandage or tape
● Follow the manufacturer's instructions when using a dressing or technology
● Assess comfort of intervention and/or dressing/bandage applied after the procedure
● Ongoing evaluation and modification of the management plan and treatment intervention is essential as wounds change over time
● More advanced, non-pharmacological techniques that require specialist training or skilled personnel, such as the use of hypnosis or therapeutic touch, can be considered

Box 10.1: Questions to assess character of pain

Does the patient have background and/or incident pain?

Quality:

❖ Describe the pain or soreness in your wound at rest. Is the pain aching or throbbing (likely to be nociceptive pain), or sharp, burning, or tingling (likely to be neuropathic pain)?

Location:

❖ Where is the pain? Is it limited to the immediate area of the wound or do you feel it in the surrounding area? Consider using body map

Triggers:

❖ What makes the pain worse? Does touch, pressure, movement, positioning, interventions, day versus night trigger pain?

Reducers:

❖ What makes the pain better? Do analgesia, bathing, leg elevation, etc help to relieve pain?

❖ Does the patient experience pain during or after dressing-related procedures?

Quality:

❖ Describe the pain the last time your dressing was removed

Location:

❖ Where was the pain? Was it limited to the immediate area of the wound or did you feel it in the surrounding area?

Triggers:

❖ What part of the procedure was most painful, eg. dressing removal, cleansing, and dressing reapplication?

❖ Application, having the wound exposed?

Reducers:

❖ What helped to reduce the pain, eg. time out, slow removal of dressing, removing the dressing yourself, etc?

Timing:

❖ How long did it take for the pain to resolve after the procedure?

WUWHS Consensus Document: Minimising pain
at wound dressing-related procedures, 2004

The WUWHS document offers the most comprehensive resource on pain management in wound-related pain from an overall perspective; several other documents were also published in the same year. The Best Practice Statement, 'Minimising Trauma and Pain in Wound Management' (Wounds UK Ltd, 2004) and 'Issues in paediatric wound care. Minimising trauma and pain' (endorsed by the Tissue Viability Nurses Association [TVNA]) are both documents that are relevant to day-to-day practice. These documents provide clear guidance to practitioners in the UK drawing upon the previous EWMA and WUWHS Documents. The documents cover the same ground as the papers previously reviewed in this chapter, and provide the same information in relation to the global perspectives of wound pain. However, in the UK Best Practice Statement, the authors recognise the need for practitioners to consider pain before the dressing change, at the dressing change, and between dressing changes. These assessments are recommended in conjunction with an assessment of the patient's global pain. This is particularly important where the patient experiences pain between dressing changes, as successful management would require a global perspective of the patient's pain. Statements 1, 2 and 3 cover the preparation, activity and evaluation of a dressing change procedure in a structured format, providing clear statements and rationale for action. The wound specific statements produced in *Boxes 10.2, 10.3,* and *10.4* (Best Practice Statement Minimising Trauma and Pain in Wound Management, 2004), produce aetiology specific treatment statements that will assist practitioners in their clinical decision-making.

'Issues in Paediatric Wound Care Minimising Trauma and Pain' (2004) follows the same process as the Wounds UK document, and uses an advisory group approach to produce a document that concentrates on paediatric wound care. The identification of the challenges associated with dealing with this client group are best shown in the way that treatment recommendations and options are made in differing age groups. The developmental changes through which children pass, from infancy to adulthood, are grouped into sections by age that ultimately dictate treatment suggestions.

The explanations of the differences in paediatric skin and the major causes of wounds in this group are given in *Box 10.5*.

Box 10.2: Statement — wound specific

Statement	Reason for statement	How to demonstrate statement is being achieved
Superficial wounds		
The pain associated with superficial wounds, such as donor sites and abrasions, when clean of infection, can be reduced by the application of a moist wound healing environment	Appropriate dressing selection can, in itself, be a useful pain management strategy	❖ There is evidence in the health records of the individual with a wound that the dressing selection reflects the potential for pain reduction
Radiotherapy wounds		
Radiotherapy treatment can cause heat, burning and localised erythema to the area receiving treatment which requires local management	Radiotherapy treatment and associated skin changes may cause pain to the individual	There is evidence in the health records of the individual that: • a thorough assessment of pain using a recognised tool has been carried out • that staff act upon individual components of the pain assessment • medication or other methods of pain relief are recorded with outcome measures
Due to the effects of radiotherapy, the tissue can become very friable and at increased risk of trauma	Trauma to the area receiving radiotherapy can occur, and should be avoided where possible and minimised where appropriate	❖ Where an area has received radiotherapy the use of tapes and adhesives should be avoided ❖ Evidence shows that where skin is dry and intact, bland moisturisers should be used ❖ Dressings which are likely to adhere or cause trauma to the wound bed should be avoided ❖ Treatment and management of radiotherapy wounds should be based on local/national practice guidelines

Box 10.3: Statement — wound specific

Statement	Reason for statement	How to demonstrate statement is being achieved
Fungating wounds		
Due to the actual disease process, wound pain can occur	Individuals with fungating wounds can have increased pain due to the ongoing disease process	There is evidence in the health records of the individual with a wound that: • a full assessment of the individual's wound pain, and emotional status has been carried out • staff act on individual components of the pain and wound assessment • wound dressings have been selected following full wound assessment and are based on each individual's symptoms • pain management strategies have been recorded with outcome measures
Trauma to wound bed or peri-wound area may be caused by traumatic dressing changes	Trauma to the wound and peri-wound area can result in pain, skin breakdown and increased risk of infection	❖ There is evidence in the health records of the individual that a full assessment has been completed ❖ Dressing selection reflects careful consideration of potential problems of adherence and trauma ❖ Dressing changes should be kept to a minimum to avoid wound bed trauma, considering individual preferences ❖ Dressing products which are likely to adhere to the wound bed should be avoided ❖ Dressings which function by causing trauma to the wound bed should not be used ❖ Where fragile skin is present in the peri-wound area, skin barriers should be considered to reduce the potential trauma of adhesion or individual sensitivity

Box 10.4: Statement — wound specific

Statement	Reason for statement	How to demonstrate statement is being achieved
Pressure ulcers		
Superficial pressure ulcers require management to prevent further wound trauma from friction	Superficial pressure ulcers, particularly on the heel and sacrum, are likely to be subjected to repeated force from friction	❖ Where appropriate, pressure ulcers will be treated with dressing products which reduce the impact of friction on the wound bed and peri-wound area
Leg ulcers		
Individuals with a painful leg ulcer will have a comprehensive assessment in line with local guidelines to establish the cause of the ulcer and the pain	Pain in leg ulcers can be caused by a variety of underlying medical conditions which require diagnosis and specialist referral	❖ The health records will record a full leg ulcer assessment (in line with local/national guidelines), and appropriate specialist referral where required
The peri-wound area of a leg ulcer should be protected from exudate to prevent skin trauma	Exudate, which is not managed effectively, can result in trauma to the skin, causing breakdown and increased pain	❖ Individuals with a leg ulcer producing exudate will have effective dressing selection (in line with local/national guidelines), which reduces the risk of peri-wound trauma
Superficial wounds		
Cavity wounds must not be packed or loosely filled with dressing products likely to adhere to the wound bed	Cavity wounds packed or loosely filled with dressing materials likely to adhere to the wound bed will cause unnecessary wound bed trauma and pain	❖ Dressing materials which are likely to adhere to the wound bed resulting in trauma and pain must not be used to pack or loosely fill surgical cavity wounds

Box 10.5: Differences in paediatric skin and the major wound causes

Paediatric skin

❖ Although the epidermal layer of the skin is structurally and functionally immature, in premature infants there is rapid postnatal maturation in the first week or two of life

❖ The epidermal thickness of a newborn is similar to that of an adult, but it is not as effective a barrier to transcutaneous water loss.

❖ The dermis of a newborn is 60% as thick and does not mature fully until about 6 months, making infant skin potentially vulnerable to trauma (excoriation, tearing and/or blistering)

❖ Throughout childhood and adolescence, there are further complex changes to the skin's characteristics, including thickening of the dermis and increased activity of sebaceous glands and hair follicles

❖ Tissue growth/regeneration is significantly faster in most children compared to adults, for example:
  • fibroblasts are present in greater numbers
  • collagen and elastic are produced more rapidly
  • granulation tissue forms more quickly
  • scars may not lengthen at the same rate of growth

Paediatric wounds:

There are two main categories of wounds that occur in infants and children, namely:

❖ **Acute:** traumatic, surgical (eg. abrasions, bites, amputations, scalds, thermal, chemical or radiation burns)

❖ **Chronic:** congenital abnormalities (eg. haemangioma), genetically-determined skin diseases (eg. epidermolysis bullosa), pressure ulcers, leg ulcers (eg. sickle cell disease), skin ulceration (caused by meningitis and dermatological conditions), malignant/fungating wounds

Issues in Paediatric Wound Care. Minimising Trauma and Pain, 2004

The main objective of this publication is to provide practical wound management guidance for healthcare professionals caring for paediatric patients. It is based on the clinical experience of the expert independent advisory group.

The major sections in the rest of the document on pain recognition, assessment and management, alongside the information related to dressing procedures, build further on the information in all of the previous publications. The main recommendations for treatment in this patient group are given in *Box 10.6*.

Box 10.6: Specific advice for different age groups

Infants aged 0–5 years
- Use a full-hand bandage for hand or finger injuries, as infants and children may suck their fingers and choke if the dressing comes off
- Skin fragility is less of an issue beyond 6 months of age but, before this age, a safe, atraumatic dressing, that will not damage fragile skin, should be selected
- To minimise the child's anxiety:
  - complete the procedure as quickly and as safely as possible
  - provide continual reassurance and distraction
  - cut and prepare dressings beforehand, and approach the child with the pre-prepared dressing

Children aged 6–11 years
- If the child wants to participate, involve them in the procedure:
  - allow a choice of dressings
  - allow them to play with the dressings, putting them on dolls, etc
  - always tell them what you are doing and do not mislead them when estimating levels of pain

Children aged 12–18 years
- The need for shower-proof dressings becomes more apparent for this age group, as regular showering becomes commonplace
- If they want to participate, teach them how to remove/replace dressings appropriately
- Patient advice leaflets and information may be useful, as they will increasingly take on board healing information and the rationale behind how the dressing works. Older children may also wish to read and understand about the dressings for themselves

---

Issues in Paediatric Wound Care. Minimising Trauma and Pain, 2004

The specialist issue of neonatal wound care was addressed by another advisory group and published in 2005 as, 'Issues in Neonatal Wound Care. Minimising Trauma and Pain. A report from an independent advisory group'. This document gives good guidance for dealing with the specialist needs of this client group. The major points are outlined in *Table 10.4*. The contents and recommendations all need to be viewed in relation to the opening paragraph on neonatal skin (*Box 10. 7*).

Box 10.7: Neonatal skin

Epidermal development is complete by the end of the second trimester of pregnancy. However, before 28 weeks gestation, the skin is thin and poorly keratinised. As a consequence, the barrier function of the skin is minimal and exposes the premature infant to:

- high transepidermal water loss (can be 10 times greater compared with an infant born at term)
- risk of excessive heat loss (skin is constantly damp due to water loss)
- increased potential for absorption of chemicals through the skin
- increased risk of iatrogenic tissue damage.

Unlike the epidermis, the dermis is not fully developed until after birth. Even at full-term, the dermis of a new-born is only 60% as thick as it is in adult skin. The fibrils connecting the epidermis and dermis are reduced in number and more widely spaced in neonatal skin, making it vulnerable to shear forces and easily removed, especially by any adhesive products (epidermal stripping). Subcutaneous fat is evident, but not fully thickened in pre-term infants.

At 24 weeks gestation, the skin appears moist, shiny and red due to the lack of subcutaneous fat between the dermis and muscle tissue.

Most importantly, exposure of the neonatal skin to air accelerates maturation. No matter how premature the infant, within 2 weeks the skin will have developed to the same extent as that of a full-term infant.

Issues in Neonatal Wound Care. Minimising Trauma and Pain, 2005

Table 10.4: Types of wounds and guidance by type

Epidermal stripping

Handling	Handle with extreme care, rings can cause damage
Removal of adhesive tapes used to secure tubes/lines	Avoid products that bond to the skin. Secure intravenous cannulae with clear, sterile film dressings, which allow monitoring of the site so that frequent removal is unnecessary. An alcohol-free skin barrier film may reduce skin stripping on removal of film dressings. Mepiform® (soft silicone dressing) is useful as a tape, particularly for those with blistering disorders, eg. epidermolysis bullosa. Use Velcro® strapping for splints, instead of tape

Pressure ulcers

Tubing	Avoid the infant lying on tubes or cannula wings
Saturation probes, if not re-sited often enough. Nasal septum, if receiving nasal continuous positive airway pressure (CPAP)	Re-site sensors/probes every 3–4 hours, or more frequently if required for very pre-term babies Consider the use of a protective dressing under cannula wings and ET tubes
Oedemateous babies* and failure to loosen tapes/clothing	Loosen tapes/clothes when baby is becoming oedematous *Oedema can occur post delivery (often a few days after birth), and in pre-terms ventilated for respiratory distress syndrome (RDS)

Extravasation injuries

Infusion irritates vein causing vasoconstriction and swelling at cannula site and surrounding tissue	Careful siting of lines/tubes (refer to local policy for guidance) Identified line usually dedicated central (caffeine, TPN, glucose > 10% should go into central line — but not always possible, may have to use a deep vein)
Cannula tip dislodges or punctures vein	Minimise risk by having good visibility of the cannula site
Device or needle poorly secured	Secure lines with transparent film dressings, allowing good observation
Obstruction of tip caused by fibrin, thrombus	Inspect lines frequently for signs of injury
Cannulae left in place too long	Median life span of IV cannulae is 36 hours

'Pain at wound dressing-related procedures: a template for assessment' (Hollinworth, 2005, available online at: http://www.worldwidewounds. com/2005/august/Hollinworth/Framework-Assessing-Pain-Wound-Dressing-Related.html) brings much of the work in the previous documents together, and proposes an assessment form to address the situation associated with pain at dressing-related procedures.

The assessment is complex in nature, with no background to wound pain or pain assessment, and may be a tool for experienced practitioners, or those working at specialist level. Personal experience and extensive consultation with pain specialists indicate that a simple assessment, with an intervention that is monitored to reduce pain, is the most appropriate for everyday practice, moving on to more experienced levels as interventions are explored and discarded.

Conclusion

The issue of pain in wound management has been extensively explored in a series of comprehensive documents over the past four years. The major focus in the early literature was related to procedural pain and efforts to avoid it. Pain in the wider context is an issue that affects patients with chronic wounds throughout their everyday existence, having a debilitating effect on quality of life. The main theme of the documents reviewed is that of accepting that pain is a problem, and assessing for and addressing the problem.

A means of addressing the problem, not just at dressing-related procedures, is promoted in the WUWHS document with the assumption that all wounds are painful. This approach is similar to that of the universal precautions in infection control: if the assumption is that a wound is painful, then simple and effective assessment tools that are easily used in everyday practice to assess pain should be a goal of practice.

The issue of pain in wound management is well addressed in the literature and with good consensus documents for guidance; the challenge now must be to see pain addressed in everyday practice and for the literature to start to reflect the improvements in quality of life for patients that this will surely bring.

References

European Wound Management Association (EWMA) (2002) *Position Document: Pain at wound dressing changes.* Medical Education Partnership Ltd, London

Hofman D, Lindholm C, Arnold F *et al* (1997) Pain in venous leg ulcers. *J Wound Care* 6: 222–4

Hollinworth H (2005) Pain at wound dressing-related procedures: a template for assessment. Available online at: www.worldwidewounds. com/2005/august/Hollinworth/Framework-Assessing-Pain-Wound_ Dressing-Related.html (accessed 3 April, 2006)

Independent advisory group (2004) *Best Practice Statement. Minimising Trauma and Pain in Wound Management.* Available online at: www.wounds-uk.com

Independent advisory group (2005) *Issues in Neonatal Wound Care. Minimising Trauma and Pain.* Sponsored by an educational grant from The Tendra Academy, Mölnlycke Health Care. Available online at: www.tendra.com

Independent multidisciplinary advisory group (2004) *Issues in Paediatric Wound Care. Minimising Trauma and Pain.* Sponsored by an educational grant from The Tendra Academy, Mölnlycke Health Care. Available online at: www.tendra.com

Krasner D (1998) Painful venous leg ulcers: themes and stories about living with the pain and suffering. *J Wound Ostomy Continence Nurs* 25(3): 158–68

Moffatt CJ, Franks PJ, Hollinworth H (2002) Understanding wound pain and trauma: an international perspective. EWMA Position Document (2002) *Pain at Wound Dressing Changes.* Medical Education Partnership, London

Noonan L, Burge SM (1998) Venous leg ulcers: is pain a problem? *Phlebology* 13: 14–19

Reddy M, Kohr R, Queen D, Keast D, Sibbald RG (2003) Practical treatment of wound pain and trauma: a patient-centered approach. An overview. *Ostomy/Wound Management* 49(4 Suppl):2–15

Rook JL (1996) Wound care pain management. *Adv Wound Care* 9(6)

Wong DL, Hockenberry-Eaton M, Wilson D, Winklestein ML, Schwartz P (2001) *Wong's Essentials of Pediatric Nursing.* 6th edn. Mosby, St Louis: 1301

World Union of Wound Healing Societies (2004) *Principles of Best Practice: Minimising pain at wound dressing-related procedures. A consensus document.* Available online at: www.wuwhs.org/pdf/consensus_eng.pdf

INDEX